To Dear friends
with my best wishes

George Abawi
March 2005

MW01289512

George M. Abouna
The History of a Pioneer in
Transplant Surgery

by

Samir Johna

Associate Clinical Professor of Surgery

Loma Linda University School of Medicine

Attending Surgeon

Southern California Permanente Medical Group

authorHOUSE

1663 LIBERTY DRIVE, SUITE 200
BLOOMINGTON, INDIANA 47403
(800) 839-8640
www.authorhouse.com

© 2004 Samir Johna
All Rights Reserved.

No part of this book may be reproduced, stored in a retrieval system, or transmitted by any
means without the written permission of the author.

First published by AuthorHouse 07/30/04

ISBN: 1-4184-8060-6 (sc)

Library of Congress Control Number: 2004095973

Printed in the United States of America
Bloomington, Indiana

This book is printed on acid-free paper.

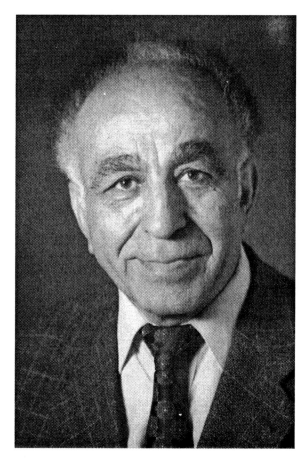

George M. Abouna, MD, MS, FRCS, FRCS(C),

FACS, FRSM, FICS

Dedication

I dedicate this book to my wife Layla, and my daughter Kristin for donating the time they deserve, for me to be able to complete this work. Without their support, this work would have not seen the light.

Acknowledgements

I have been most fortunate in having the tremendous support of Dr. George Abouna and his family, more so by his daughter Linda. I would like to thank those who worked behind the scenes to make ends meet. To name a few, the honorable Ralph Klein, the Premier of Alberta, Canada; Mr. R. Sykes, the former Mayor of Calgary; Dr. Ghazi Karim; Donald Moores, MD; David Welsh, MD; Moshe Schien, MD, and Makram Murad-al-Shaikh.

Contents

Foreword

One Saturday afternoon, on October 25th, 2003, I hit the road to San Diego, California, to meet Dr. George Abouna, who was on a visit to his son's family. On the way there, I had no idea how I was going to start my interview. A few days earlier, and for the first time in over two decades, we had met at the American College of Surgeons Clinical Congress in Chicago, where he had handed me a brief case loaded with documents that he had collected over the years from different places where he had visited or worked.

Because I was fascinated by his contributions to surgery and his surgical education for the Middle East, he has been my role model ever since I was in medical school, especially given that he comes from the same ethnic background as I. George is a Chaldean, and I am an Assyrian[1]. We both belong to one nation erroneously named differently, and to a small Christian minority that is still struggling for existence in its own homeland—a nation forced to live like nomads for decades to survive the atrocities it was subjected to. For such a nation, a man like George represents a triumph against all adversities and a sure sign that it is still viable.

In San Diego, I was welcomed by George, a pleasant gentleman in his late sixties, on whom the years had left obvious marks. His black hair had been replaced by gray, and his hairline had recessed backwards to show more of his wrinkled forehead. His lower eyelids seemed to be burdened with two small eye sacs. Although his eyebrows had remained high, they had turned gray and lost their luster. I saw many changes in his physical appearance but, luckily, no real change in his soul.

I started my interview by simply asking George to narrate what he remembers from his early childhood to the present day. For the fear of my memory not coming to my rescue, I asked for a permission to tape the interview. After a couple of hours, I realized that my task would take more than just one session. Over the following few months, we had other

---

[1] **Who Are We?**
Why our nation today assumes so many different names is shrouded in mystery. However, historical facts support that Assyrians, Chaldeans, Syriacs, Aramaics, Jacobites, and whatever else that might be out there, are nothing but one nation that has been divided over the centuries by the evolving religious denominations.

meetings, some of which were conducted over the phone, not only with him but also with other people in his life.

I realize that it is a different time not only in Iraq but also in every country in which George had worked. Nevertheless, I was able to compile enough information—often supported by documents—to paint my portrait of George Abouna and his life: the life of a man for whom my nation and I carry a lot of respect. I hope that it reflects enough colors for all of us to enjoy.

The Author

Introduction

It is a fact of life that all great men start out unrecognized and often underestimated long before they make their mark in life. The general custom, then, is for those failed to recognize the seeds of excellence in the distant past to claim that 'I knew him when...' But there are other cases, too, when some traumatic experience forces the recognition of outstanding qualities perhaps earlier than they would have been generally recognized.

Such is the case of George Abouna, I think: for when he lived in Calgary, Alberta, in the foothills of the Western Canadian Plains almost thirty years ago, he was forced to defend both his personal integrity and his professional competence in the face of discreditable attack based on outright lies that were themselves based on deliberately falsified records. What is worse, far worse for a young doctor, is the fact that the very university and medical establishment that he should have been able to look to for support were the source of the attack.

What is the point of raking up a sad story from more than a quarter of a century ago; other places, other times? The point is that adversity shows the quality of the man. Intolerance and injustice have destroyed many good people, but they made George Abouna all the stronger in his convictions, without which he could never have achieved world-wide recognition in both Eastern and Western circles, where medical excellence is understood and celebrated. George Abouna's experience in Alberta is, literally, a profile in courage; one that plays a part in the making of a man.

The story is simple although the playing-out of it isn't-more to come later. Our new university and its new Faculty of Medicine needed to improve the results of its transplant program, then regarded as "showcase" surgery, a source of prestige and evidence of our maturity. The existing program boasted successful but limited procedures. The opportunities offered in a new system attracted Dr. Abouna, who knew little or nothing about Canadian government-run socialized medicine, and the politics and the stifling bureaucracy that go with the state control everywhere in the socialized world. He was about to learn a hard lesson.

Within fairly a short time, it was noticed that morbidity and mortality rates in the transplant program had improved; and the contrast with the immediate past was uncomfortable for our medical establishment. The "team system" they had adopted made no one person responsible for results, but it didn't seem to work well for patients; while George Abouna's taking over direct control of all phases of transplant treatment, with obvious success, aroused feelings of jealousy, as subsequent events seemed to show. Here was a setting for conflict. The new man from somewhere else, because of the very success he had been asked to produce, was a serious embarrassment to the local university establishment.

In due course, George Abouna's medical privileges were suspended on the grounds of what later turned out to be falsified medical records. He appeared to be denied the normal due process, and it was clearly hoped that he would go away.

But George Abouna didn't go quietly. Finding no support inside the system, he went outside it. He went to the news media and enlisted then-television reporter, Ralph Klein, who is now premier of Alberta, and myself-then Calgary's mayor, both of whom worked to get him a fair hearing. It proved impossible to get a fair hearing from the political establishment of the time, as it was for the medical and university establishment; and there was no alternative but the courts, and so there he went with the assistance of one of the outstanding lawyers of his time, the late Mr. Justice Ross McBain.

Although the legal process took several years of anxiety and costs, George Abouna won hands-down and he was awarded heavy damages in a decision that recognized clearly the wrongs done to him, and condemned unreservedly the behavior of the university and the medical staff involved. The findings of the court that medical records had been falsified to misrepresent Dr. Abouna's performance was humiliating, and it should have been crushing in any system devoted to the ethical practice of medicine.

No such victory, overwhelming as it eventually was, can make for popularity in any medical establishment, however, and the fact that the Canadian Association of University Teachers (CAUT) blacklisted Calgary's university for years after did not help but served rather to rub salt into the wounds.

George Abouna left Calgary for greater things, with his reputation for integrity and professional competence intact. The losers were, of course, the western Canadians who had lost their access to one of the finest transplant surgeons in the world as patients, and as medical students. Losses such as these are measured in lives lost, and those can never be recovered.

As for me, with my small part in helping George Abouna get what passes for justice in our part of the world, I can feel privileged to have known him. I only hope that the purgatory he passed through in Alberta contributed in some positive way to his great achievements of the later years. I am sure it did.

Rod Sykes
Former Mayor of Calgary
Alberta, Canada
May 24th, 2004

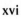

Chapter I
Prologue
Elkosh, Iraq
1927–1939

It was just another day in Elkosh, a small town in the heartland of Assyria, the cradle of civilization, when a young villager, Mansour Abouna, found his better half, Rachel, who chose to give her heart and soul to the Abouna family. Like many newlywed couples, they were blessed by the arrival of their first-born child, a baby girl whom they named Warda. Almost five years later, on April 5th, 1933, their joy was compounded by the arrival of a second child, a baby boy they named Gerjis (George). At the time, nothing seemed special about George; he was just another child born to a typical Christian family. But George lived to beat all the odds and managed to carve his name in the books of medicine through his lifelong achievements in one of the most innovative and promising fields for mankind—the surgery of organ transplantation. But wait! I am getting ahead of myself in narrating his story.

Elkosh is located 35 miles north of the ancient city of Nineveh (one of the four capitals of the Assyrian Empire)[2], in the northern part of present-day Iraq. The history of Elkosh goes back to as early as, and probably before, the days of Nahum the prophet, around the seventh century B.C. (also known as Nahum the Elkoshite in the Old Testament). It is believed that the town took its name from the Assyrian "Eal-Kash," which means "The Grand God." The Assyrians used to bring this god of theirs to the resort town of Elkosh every April 1st, when they celebrated the beginning of their new year.

Elkosh was among a few other towns in the region to accept Christianity early on. Although Edessa is believed to be the first Assyrian city to have done so in 32 A.D. when the apostle Addai was sent by the disciple Judas Thomas, as promised by the Lord. Elkosh soon followed in the footsteps of Edessa, and since then, Elkosh has been the home of many prominent convents and holy sites such as the convents of Rabban Hirmiz, Mar

---

[2] **Ancient capitals of Assyria;**
Nimrud (Kalhu, Calah); Niniveh; Dur-Sharrukin (Khorsabad); and Ashur.

Matay, Mart Maryam, and Mar Qardakh and the tomb of Nahum, to name a few, and the seat for several Assyrian Patriarchs of the Ancient Church of the East (also known as the Nestorian Church)[3].

George and his sister Warda were born to a small farming family that lived a simple life, using their own resources. The average family of the time lived in a single room typically built from rocks or dried mud bricks. There would have been virtually no furniture other than the bedding, which was rolled up against the walls when not in use, and some earthen utensils and cooking pots. Each family lived on their local produce of cereals, fruits, and vegetables and on products from their flocks. In fact even today the best watermelons in Iraq are grown in Elkosh! Hardly anything was wasted from their animals; the meat and dairy products were the backbone of their nutrition. Feathers, wool, and skins were used for clothing and bedding. Even the manure was turned into cakes to be used for an energy source, if it was not used as fertilizer. With scant opportunity for or awareness of proper education and schooling, the children usually followed in the footsteps of their parents. Boys learned farming, while girls learned how to clean, cook, and take care of the rest of the household, a long, difficult, hands-on training process to become good homemakers when the time came for them to be married. For the most part, people were content with this way of life, because they knew no other. But right around the time that George was born, Elkosh, like many other Christian villages in Iraq, was about to face yet another example of human savagery, when innate jealousy and the struggle for power and possession wash all ideals away. It was the irony of fate for the Assyrians to become a minority in their own homeland—a country full of fanatics, by all accounts. The Assyrian villages were scattered among, and surrounded by, larger Arab and Kurdish villages. This often created an atmosphere of tension between the Assyrians and many of their neighbors. George was only four months old when the Iraqi government, under King Ghazi, massacred innocent Assyrian civilians in many northern villages of Iraq. The massacre of Sumail near Duhok is only one example. Some survivors still remember Captain Ismael Abbawi of the Mosul Police taking the lead in shooting

---

[3] **The Nestorian Church**

The Assyrian church (Ancient Church of the East) was called the Nestorian Church in the 4th century after its patriarch Nestorios. In 431 AD, the Catholic Church through its council in Ephesus had deposed Nestorios because of what was considered heretical doctrines by his denial of the complete mergence of the divine and human natures in the person of the Christ. He asserted that Mary, the mother of Christ, should not be called the mother of God. The Assyrians have been called Nestorians eversince.

and stabbing several hundred elderly people, women, and children on August 7th, 1933[4], with the help and instigation of many locals under the leadership of General Bakir Sidqi of the Iraqi army. The ordeal was not over until the Assyrian Patriarch, Mar Shimun, was exiled to Cyprus on August 18th, 1933. The toll of Assyrian lives reached several thousands, along with major property losses caused by destruction, confiscation, and looting.

In his quest for a better life and a decent future for his children, George's father, Mansour, moved with his family to the capital city of Baghdad when George was only five or six years old. They left behind loved ones and their vivid memories in the search for new hope in a land of uncertainty.

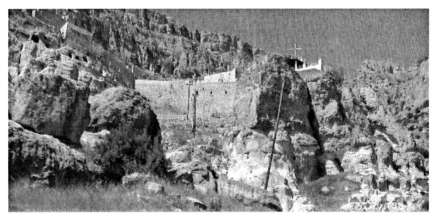

Rabban Hirmiz Monastery, Elkosh (Courtesy of Firas Jatou)

---

[4] **The Assyrian Martyr Day;**
In memory of those massacred, the Assyrian communities all over the world observe the Assyrian Martyr Day on August 7th of every year.

Chapter 2
Moving to Baghdad
1939

It was a sad day for the Abouna family when they left Elkosh. It never occurred to them that they would miss their home before they even left! The long journey to Baghdad was set in motion. Under the morning blue sky, fresh blossoms scented the soft winds over the green prairies between Elkosh and Mosul. Another look at the ruins of Nineveh took Mansour centuries into the dark past. Overwhelmed by emotion, for him it seemed as if history was repeating itself! Centuries before, his predecessors had been forced to escape into the mountains when Nineveh was ransacked and destroyed, leaving nothing behind but a few silent artifacts that could not attest to the rest of the world the glory they once had[5].

Mansour knew that the hardest days were still ahead of him. Along with his wife and his two children, he had to face the uncertainty in a place where he had little help, if any. In the midst of thinking, he reached out for his tobacco pouch, ready to roll a cigarette. He lit the cigarette and took a deep sigh. Looking through the windows he exhaled as if he was trying to blow away all of his worries! The smile on the faces of his children made him keep his worries to himself. He tried to escape thinking about his looming problems as he attempted to focus on the scenery along the route. Unfortunately, there was not much to see! Most of the land south of Mosul is dry and relies heavily on rain. Once the rainy season is over, the land looks like a flat yellow basin, with some hills here and there but no signs of life other than a few small Arab villages scattered along the way, some of which have resting-places for travelers. He could not help but to think about the possibility of failing in his endeavor. Finally, he came to terms with himself.

"It is not a failure if I fall, but it is a total failure if I stay where I fall. I just have to pick myself up and keep going," he thought.

---

[5] **The fall of the Assyrian Empire;**
In 612 BC, Niniveh was ransacked by the combined forces of the Babylonians and Medes. Haran, the last Assyrian stronghold, was taken in 610 BC, ending the Assyrian empire.

It was late in the afternoon when the Abouna family made it to Baghdad, a totally different environment compared with the small towns and villages they had lived in. The city had new buildings with modern architectural designs, public squares, statures, neat gardens and wide, clean, paved streets. Stores were busy with customers; many of whom were dressed in western styles. New cars zoomed all day through the streets—a sure sign of life!

Although Baghdad was trying hard to catch up with the rest of the civilized world, many scenes from the past were still evident on its streets. Transport and passenger cars pulled by horses, and in the bazaars, people, horses, donkeys, mules, and even camels mixed together! It was ironic to see clothes and shoes placed in shiny and clean glass cabinets, whereas vegetables, fruits, and dairy products were placed outside along with animal carcasses hanging outside butcher shops exposed to dust and all kinds of insects (a common practice in all third-world countries). No wonder infectious diseases were so prevalent.

A few friends and relatives offered some support and welcomed the Abouna family until they were able to rent their own place. Needless to say, Mansour had to find some means of making a living in a hurry. They settled in an overpopulated neighborhood of Baghdad called Al-Sinak, off Al-Rashid Street at the Risafa bank of the Tigris River. This was the commercial and industrial area of the capital, where the prospects for employment were much higher. As expected, only a few families could afford to rent a house on their own. It was common practice to see many poor families, particularly immigrants from rural areas, sharing larger houses in order to cut down on their expenses. Many of these houses had a traditional look in terms of their architectural design, having balustrades known as "Shanashil."

Each family would live in two rooms or so with only primitive furniture. The rest of the household facilities were usually shared among all of the residents. It is interesting to note that, even today, when the weather gets hot during the summer, people carry their bedding up to sleep on the roofs! Modern utilities were virtually nonexistent. A very few families owned refrigerators and air cooling devices such as fans, swamp coolers, and air conditioners. Most people used iceboxes or some natural means to temper the weather or to cool down their drinking water. The water was kept in a large conical cistern—the Hib—which was made from baked clay. It held between 20 and 30 gallons of water. The evaporation of water filtered to the outside surface of the Hib through its tiny pores leads to a temperature drop and a cooling effect. A thirsty person would dip a metal bowl—a Tasa—into the Hib to get water. A similar utensil albeit smaller—the Tunga—holds a half a gallon of water or so and was usually carried to other places when needed.

Except for a few cinemas, entertainment was limited to social gatherings among family and friends. Typically, the children played in the streets; women took turns gathering in their homes for chatting, and the men spent their free time gathering at small local coffee shops—Gahwa—to smoke tobacco in water pipes—Nargila—and to drink coffee, tea, and other herbal drinks. Gahwa provided some entertainment as well, such as dominos, backgammon, and playing cards. Some of them used to hold small local musical concerts—Chalghi—where folk singing—Al-Maqam—took place. Other Gahwas were better equipped and had gramophones for playing music. Although electricity was available in the capital, it was not until some years later that radio and television stations were established. Radio and television sets were commodities owned only by those who were wealthy or by some Gahwas. Although it was less than optimal, this new life was all that Mansour could provide for his family; he hoped that it would be a good enough start for his children in a city that certainly had more opportunities than Elkosh.

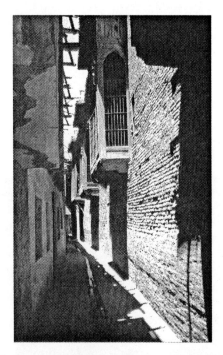

A typical alley in Baghdad at the turn of the last century

Chapter 3
Early Years in School
1939–1951

The two new kids on the block, Warda and George seemed to adjust quite well to their new lifestyle. It was not long before they made friends in the neighborhood with whom they enjoyed playing. Unlike Warda, who had had her first few years of schooling in the north, George was excited to discover the new world of school, the promised land where he could satisfy his nagging eagerness to learn.

Classes in the public schools of Baghdad were taught in Arabic, a different language from George's native tongue. For him, starting his first grade in Arabic did not seem to be a problem at all. Before he started, he had learned many words and phrases from his friends. Once he picked up

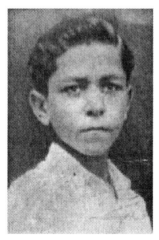

George Abouna- early childhood

the Arabic alphabet, he was well on the way toward excelling in his class.

Going through the same process myself in 1965, I could not imagine what it had been like as a first grader three decades earlier. The limited resources of the pupils and the public schools made it very hard to carry on an effective educational program. As such, the burden of learning fell mostly on the pupils and their families rather than the educational system itself. Except for a decent curriculum, teaching techniques were primitive, and laboratories and teaching aids were almost unheard of. There were some cruel punishments that were justified by school officials as means of discipline. Verbal abuse, embarrassment, and even the physical abuse of those children were everyday practice and were viewed as necessary by their teachers. Missing homework or the inability to answer a question correctly were sure tickets to such a fate!

But for George and many other bright students, this hostile environment was not looked at as a hurdle but rather as an impetus for them to continue the hard and long journey to success! After all, this was where George learned reading, writing, arithmetic, science, society, religion, and some basics about art. At the end of his sixth year, he was ready for the first national examinations. It was no surprise that he excelled and passed on to the next level of education, intermediate school, with flying colors.

It was around this time that Warda became aware of the financial burdens on her father. She believed that by going into an accelerated path of education she would guarantee a decent job through which she could help with expenses. Warda chose to go into an integrated nursing program, a booming profession that was not yet popular among women in Iraq. This proved to be a smart move on her part, as she became capable of providing the much-needed help for her family in a short period of time. In addition to financial security, for George it was an eye-opening experience to see his sister pursue a career helping the poor and the sick. And who knows how much of an influence Warda's profession left on George's subconscious mind in choosing his future career?

The next three years at the Mansour Intermediate School, in Hafidh Al-Qadhi neighborhood of Baghdad, were an opportunity for George to solidify his basic knowledge in science, mathematics, history, and languages. Life seemed to be 'business as usual," except for some trivial instability caused by the public unrest and insurgency against the government of Baghdad. This was the time when the Middle East was ravaged by the looming problems in Palestine and the declaration of the state of Israel. The public always viewed the government in Baghdad as a puppet for the British Crown in taking political stances that had put the national Arabic and Islamic interests at risk. But George kept his distance from politics, simply because he believed that even discussions in those matters would only generate heat and no light! He managed to dissolve the political controversies around him and focused his attention on his education, as reflected by his high scores in his second national examination at the end of his ninth year of schooling.

Finally, George had to face the most critical stage in his pre college education: the final two years at Al-Markazia High School in the Al-Maidan neighborhood, one of the few reputable high schools still standing in Baghdad today. This was, and still is, the most stressful stage, because it is followed by the third national examinations, the scores of which dictate students' future professional life. On the basis of their scores, students are ranked, and those with higher scores are given priority in choosing their educational paths by filling the available spots.

At that time, for George it was not a question of choice but rather a question of how to get there! He had already chosen science during high school in preparation for his life's dream—to be a doctor. Growing up in a populated neighborhood in Baghdad, he saw many poor and many sick people who could not afford health care. He watched many of them falling prey to their illnesses, one after another, with very little that he could do. Out of his frustration with the status quo, he thought his services as a physician to the needy and poor could put an end to the social Darwinism so deeply entrenched in his society. It was clear to him that he had to be among the top-graduating students in high school to be able to win a seat in medical school. For him it was not an option anymore: it was necessary!

Although the first year of high school was not as stressful in general, the system at Al-Markazia High School had made this otherwise. Students were assigned to their classes according to the scores that they had received at the end of the preceding year. Those with the highest scores were assigned to class"A," whereas the less fortunate ones were assigned to class "B," and so on. That by itself put a tremendous pressure on the students because of everyone's high expectations of them.

George was assigned to class "A," along with his colleague and lifelong friend, Dr. Ghazi Karim[6]. The environment was extremely competitive at a time when they both had to work part time. Together, they were able to plan a systematic program by which every subject was given its share of attention. The curriculum was divided into sections equal to the number of hours they had to attend class. A typical after-school day would start with them going over the subjects to be covered in the next day's lectures. This ensured a better perspective and allowed them to ask intelligent

---

[6] **Ghazi A. Karim;**
Professor, Faculty of Engineering, University of Calgary, Alberta, Canada. B.Sc. (Hons.), University of Durham, England; D.I.C., Imperial College, London, England; Ph.D. (Mech. Engg.), University of London, England; and D.Sc. (Engg.), University of London, England.

questions, thus filling as many gaps as possible in their understanding of the material.

That seemed to be a wonderful plan, but there were too many hurdles in the way. For one, George, like many others, could hardly find a quiet and accessible place to study. Just like the Bedouins, he had to find his own oasis of serenity amid chaos. Oftentimes, such a place was at a friend's house, a public place, or even a Gahwa. Public libraries were scarce and were crowded when they were available. To complicate matters even more, the educational system itself did not help. All tests were based on questions that required a problem-solving approach and long essay answers rather than multiple-choice questions. When studying, students had to follow a labor-intense and time-consuming strategy that relied not only on learning and recalling the facts when needed but also on being able to express them in constructed phrases and paragraphs when writing their essays.

To help with family expenses, George managed to generate some extra income by part-time jobs on the weekends and during the long summer holidays. He was a salesperson in an antique shop, as well as a helper in one of the local churches. His entertainment was limited to watching movies at a local theatre with his friends every Thursday night. With the little extra time left, he indulged himself in some extracurricular school activities that culminated in his winning his first high-caliber award during high school.

During the final year at Al-Markazia High School, students were required to research and present an original topic as part of a competition. George had the courage to choose a subject at a point in time when very few would want to discuss it openly: to talk about women and their role in Arab society was like opening a bag of worms, but his focused research and the facts he gathered gave him the upper hand above all others in affirming his conclusions in favor of women. For that work, the minister of education in Iraq awarded George first prize.

But the moment of truth was getting closer. The scheduled third national examinations would be in mid-June, 1951. Everybody, including George, was nervous and restless. It was very hard to maintain composure knowing this was his only chance for a bright future. No exceptions were given even for illness or family emergencies! It was a very trying week indeed for patience, discipline, and self-control.

A few weeks later the examination was over and new worries replaced the old ones!

"Did I do well?"

"Will my scores be good enough for medical school?"

Too many questions with no sure answers played across his mind pending the day when the results were to be announced. Only high scores would cause his soul to blossom and allow him to catch his rainbow.

Finally, the fruits of 11 years of schooling were ripe and ready for the grand harvest! George, along with Ghazi, was announced to be among the best three graduates in the nation. This guaranteed a pass to any educational path he might pursue inside Iraq, as well as more opportunities for education abroad through scholarships fully paid by the Iraqi government. There were no words for George to express his joy and relief; he could have not asked for more.

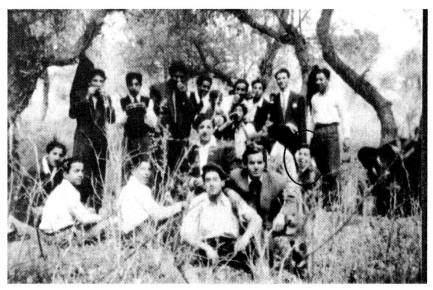

George Abouna with his high school class in a local trip

Chapter 4

College of Science & Technology, Sunderland
King's College, Newcastle-Upon-Tyne
University Of Durham
1951–1956

In the fall of 1951, George faced yet another challenge. He qualified for a college education in United Kingdom via a fully paid scholarship by the Iraqi Government. This had opened many new prospects and gave him an opportunity to discover a new world he had incessantly read about but never had the opportunity to see. A chance to learn at one of the most respective universities in United Kingdom offered immense prestige and reputation well above that of the local graduates.

To George's dismay, there were no scholarships in medicine. The government's argument was that the Royal College of Medicine in Baghdad[7] was well established and was capable of training solid physicians, so that there was no need to send students abroad. Needless to say, it was a difficult dilemma for George to choose between what he always wanted to do and the prospects of studying abroad.

George yielded to temptation and finally resolved to accept a scholarship at Durham University in mechanical engineering. The fact that he was not alone in his decision made it a little easier for him to accept reality. A few of his friends from Al-Markazia High School, including Ghazi Karim made similar decisions.

During that time, Dr. Muhammad Musaddak was the Prime Minister of Iran[8]. In 1950, and within few weeks in office, he nationalized Iran's petroleum industry, which led to a political crisis with Britain. This culminated in a severing of diplomatic ties between the two countries.

[7] **Royal College of Medicine, Baghdad, Iraq;**
Established in 1922 by the Iraqi Monarch's Chief Physician, Dr. Harry C. Sinderson.

[8] **Muhammad Musaddak (1882-1967);**
A veteran Public servant through the reign of the Persian monarchs. He was elected a prime minister who led Iran's first nationalist government in 1951. After nationalizing Iran's oil industry, his government was overthrown by a military coup that was orchestrated by CIA and British intelligence in 1953.

Because Iran produced half of the oil from Middle East at that time, the decision clearly resulted in a global energy crisis. The flight between Baghdad and England required several stops at different cities for refueling.

On October 14th, 1951 George, along with 36 other students, took off from Baghdad International Airport on the way to England. They left Baghdad in a small plane at 9:00 am heading toward Nicosia, Cyprus, where the first refueling took place. From there they flew to Athens, Greece, for the second refueling, and then on to Valletta, Malta, where the group stayed overnight in a luxurious hotel. Ghazi remembers it as quite a night, much unlike anything they had ever experienced. George and Ghazi went down to the lobby looking for something to do. They were led to a concert and then to some bars, where music and dancing were in order, which were certainly very exciting for young men raised in a totally different culture. They toured the streets of Valletta before they went back to their hotel, where they shared the same room. The following day they took off for Marseille, France, for the final refueling before they arrived in London at 3:00 pm on October 15th, 1951.

In London, Hikmat Abdul-Majeed, the Educational Attaché of the Iraqi Embassy, welcomed the students. They stayed for four nights at the Luxurious Grosvenor Hotel in Victoria, London[9]. After some errands were run and the distribution of the students to their final destination was completed, George and Ghazi, along with eight more students took a train to the northern city of Sunderland.

The local educational authorities welcomed the arriving students and took them for an overnight stay in one of the local hotels. The following morning, they were taken to some local boarding houses on the beach at 16 Roker Terrace. After 2 weeks or so, Ghazi moved out to live with a local family, whereas George stayed in his boarding house for the next four years.

Both George and Ghazi reported to the College of Science & Technology in Sunderland for their General Certificate of Education (GCE)[10]. It was a program with two levels. The first one, the ordinary level, lasted one year, during which seven courses were taken. Among others, they took basic and applied mathematics, physics, chemistry, and languages. For them, the

[9] **Grosvenor Hotel;**
Currently called the "Thistle Victoria" located on Buckingham Palace Road, Victoria, London SW1W 0SJ.
[10] **Sunderland Technical College;**
Established in 1901.

requirement of a second language was no problem! They both took Arabic. The advanced level then followed, during which they took three courses over a one-year period, thus becoming eligible to complete their degrees in engineering.

Life in Sunderland was totally different than Baghdad. The fact that neither of them had to work for a living made it easier for them to explore the local community. Certainly they had more free time on their hands for hobbies and entertainment than ever before. With such an open society, they both wished to take dancing lessons and attended classes two or three evenings a week at a small local dancing school. George, as usual, took the matter very seriously and turned out to be quite a good dancer! During a short period of time, he surprised his friends by buying his first car ever, a tiny Morris Mini. These few changes made it much easier for George to merge socially into the new society.

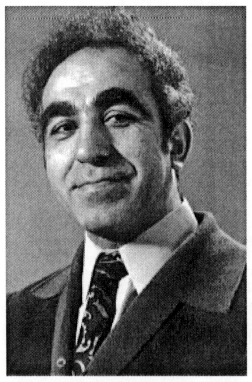

Early years in England

The advanced level year was credited as first year of engineering. Two more years were spent in studying core mechanical engineering, after which George and Ghazi passed their final tests. Then they had to spend another year, a form of internship, to be able to earn their B.Sc. degrees. They were offered a choice between doing an honor year in mechanical engineering versus taking a second major in engineering. Ghazi took the former, while George took the latter and completed a second major in electrical engineering at King's College, Newcastle-Upon-Tyne.

While during his final year at Durham University, George and Jennifer Towel got married after a couple of years of dating. Jennifer, a student of Arts at Goldsmith College of London University[11], met George during a students' work camp in northeast England. The many things they had in common turned their dreams into reality.

In 1956, George and Jennifer celebrated two exciting events: the birth of their first baby girl, Linda, and George's well-earned graduation. George was granted a B.Sc. in mechanical engineering and a B.Sc. in electrical engineering—an achievement that proved to be very handy during the years that followed.

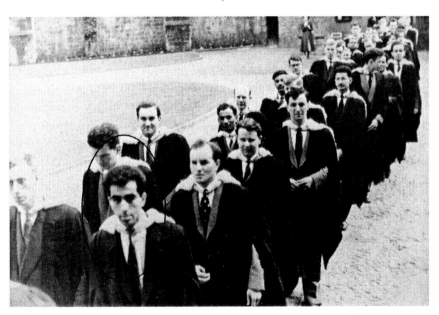

Graduation with degrees in Engineering, University of Durham

---

[11] **Goldsmith College;**
Founded in 1891 and has been part of the University of London since 1904.

Chapter 5

Back to Future

1956

His mission was accomplished, and it was time for George to go back home. After being sponsored for five years, it was time for him to give back! As expected, he would become a government employee stuck in a rather stable and prosperous job. But a worrisome question came across George's mind,

"What if I do not enjoy what I will be doing?"

He realized that going back to Baghdad meant a life sentence in engineering without parole! There would be not even a chance of a dream about his old passion; medicine. George decided to explore the possibility of being sponsored again by the Iraqi government for medical school in United Kingdom but to no avail. He tried hard to make a case by discussing the matter with the educational attaché at the Iraqi embassy in London. His requests were rejected because the Iraqi government needed him as an engineer more than as a physician.

But the depressing news was not about to make George give up easily. First, he had to find a job because no more money was coming his way, particularly given that he was responsible for a family. Jennifer did her best to help by working as an art teacher in Newcastle, but that was not enough to make ends meet. George was able to get an employment at a nuclear power plant in Stockton-on-Tees. His new job was exciting, because it allowed him to dwell on an interest of his, heat transfer, which he had developed during his years of college.

"Who knows? I might even like it!" he must have thought to himself.

George and his family might have lived very comfortably with his new career, but it was not quite the thriller he was looking for. Every time he wore his white lab coat he was reminded that he was in the wrong place! Even the long days of hard work could not make him forget. The more he tried to escape his thoughts, the more he was haunted by his oppressed desire to become a doctor. Before long George accepted once and for all that medicine was his destiny and there was no way out of it. It was a done deal and he just had to come up with some means to fund himself for the next five years through medical school.

It all started again when George wrote a letter to the Dean of the College of Medicine, University of Durham and submitted his application for admission[12]. The application was strange, yet interesting enough for the Dean to grant him an interview.

"Mr. Abouna you are now an established engineer and you could make a very comfortable living with your qualifications. Why would you want to go into this seemingly endless tunnel of medicine?" the Dean asked.

"Sir my heart is still in medicine. I wanted to be a doctor ever since I was in high school" George replied.

"To my knowledge this is almost unprecedented in UK but I promise you that we will look into it. You know there are many applicants competing with you," the Dean stated.

"One more question Mr. Abouna. You no longer have a grant. How are you going to fund yourself?" The Dean asked.

"I've got it all worked out, sir. I am going to work part time while I am in medical school. I have lined up some part-time jobs—as a lecturer at Gateshead College, as an ice-cream seller during the weekends for an Italian factory called De Maceio, as a mailman at the post office, as a waiter in a Chinese restaurant, and during Easter I will be working at a food store. Here is how much I am going to make, which I think will be enough to pay for all of my expenses" George replied.

A few weeks later George was informed that his application for medical school had been accepted!

"Mr. Abouna you have shown so much enthusiasm, perseverance, and commitment to this profession that we could not turn you down," the Dean said.

It was then, and only then, that George felt he was finally on the track to his future.

---

[12] The University of Durham College of Medicine;
Originally called the School of Medicine and Surgery and later the College of Medicine, was established in 1834.

Chapter 6

University of Durham College of Medicine

Newcastle-Upon-Tyne

1956–1961

It had been a long detour since George had graduated from high school. To say the least, he had traveled a bumpy road that taught him many lessons, perhaps the most important of which was not to settle for less than what he always wanted. The path ahead was still long and fraught with many hurdles and hardships, but, at the end of the day, he knew that someway and somehow he would be able to get there.

It was very trying to work several jobs and care for a family while studying medicine at the same time, all the more so when Judith, their second daughter, was born in 1958. It was so hard that Jennifer, along with Linda and Judith, stayed for an extended period of time in London with her parents. George worked after school and during weekends and holidays. Among all his jobs, he enjoyed selling ice cream the most. Every weekend, he would take off with a loaded truck heading toward Whitley Bay, an hour's drive from Newcastle-Upon-Tyne.

"Mom Curly is here! I want some ice cream!" many kids would scream.

The children used to call George "Curly" because of his black curly hair. They loved Curly because he always gave them larger portions of ice cream for their money. Curly enjoyed the long line of kids at his truck. He saw in their eyes his own daughters, with whom he so rarely spent time because of his busy schedule.

Another interesting job that George picked up while in his emergency room rotation was working as a waiter at the Make-way Chinese restaurant. George was on call one night when the owner of the restaurant was brought to the emergency room complaining of shortness of breath. George took such an active role in caring for the gentleman that he was offered a job! Being friendly, with a good sense of humor and a good command of the English language, he became a popular waiter in a short period of time, which bothered the other Chinese waiters.

"He is requested by too many customers and he is collecting all the tips", the waiters complained to the owner!

Despite the tremendous pressure, George enjoyed his schoolwork. The first three years in medical school were focused on basic sciences, during which he studied physics, chemistry, biochemistry, physiology, anatomy, microbiology, pathology, and pharmacology, to name but a few. The anatomy courses were the most fascinating for him. The more he dissected the cadavers, the more he appreciated the marvelous creation of God, a constellation of extremely complex organ systems so intricately orchestrated to play the symphony of life!

As an avid reader, George took every advantage of any extra time in studying and researching many topics in medicine. It was no surprise that he was among the best students in medical school, as reflected by his high scores and by his taking the challenge of submitting four projects in competition for the four endowed prizes in medicine, of which he managed to win three: the Gibb Scholarship and Prize in Pathology (1960), the Dickinson Scholarship and Prize in Surgery (1961), and the Otterson-Wood Prize in Psychological Medicine (1961), which were all awarded to him by the University of Durham. This was a win-win situation to say the least, and it opened for him a new horizon of writing and publishing his work. Equally important was that each prize paid between 100 and 150 pounds in cash, providing him and his family a much-needed financial break.

The first peer-reviewed article that George published as a medical student was in the form of a poem in which he provided a detailed description of the development of the fetal circulation. The article, "Fetal Circulation in Rythme," appeared in the *University of Durham Medical Gazette.* It was so well received by his fellow students that it was republished in the journal of the British Medical Students' Association. Then his second article came out, "Acute Pancreatitis Complicating Pregnancy," followed by a third, "Science, Medicine and Poetry." Finally, he published his fourth article in the same journal, "Arabian Contribution to Medical Science". Once again, this article was so well received in the Middle East that it was republished after expansion in the *Kuwait Medical Association Journal* in 1980.

Among these four articles, I would like to touch upon three. "Fetal Circulation in Rythme" is so interesting that I will let it speak for itself:

THE FOETAL CIRCULATION IN RYTHME

To teach and amuse are my only aims,
to skill or fame, in verse, I make no claims.
******
The life giving blood runs round every day,

19

From mother to foetus making its way.
It leaves the sponge which we call placenta
Umbilicus to Hepatis Porta.
Here it unites with the left portal vein,
Which in the liver divides once again.
But the Ductus Venosus for it made,
To fill Vena Cava Inferior
Which to the Hepar lies posterior.

Here it begins to share its crimson hue
With caval blood therein ascending blue
And enters so the right atrial cave
In streamline and not in turbulent wave;
The Oval Foramen makes now its aim,
Through caval valve, Eustachian by name.
Having entered the left atrial space
The ventricle falls with delicate pace,
Whence raised by the left ventricular beat
The arching Aorta's waiting to greet.

Oxygenated blood is meant to flow,
To the arms, neck and brain, to make them grow.
And so the pure blood swift follows its fate
Aorta, Carotids, Innominate.
The remainder of this blood now descends
To feed all the viscera it intends.

Let's now leave the pure blood and take instead
Venous fluid coming from arms and head.
From Upper Cava shoots the purple stream,
On the right A-V cusps straight as a beam,
To fill up the ventricle on the right
From whence it is pushed to another height.
Since the foetal lung is still shrunk and wet
The flowing blood is with resistance met,
So from pulmonary Trunk straight it goes:
Ductus and Aorta anastomose.

The little blood in the trunk that remains,
Through the Pulmonary Arteries drains;
Returning via Pulmonary Veins,

And so the left atrium it attains.
From Aorta blood, in oxygen low,
Flows to thorax, abdomen and below;
And from internal Iliacs passes
Through arteries to Umbilicus.
Along the tortuous cord makes its aim
Placental lakes, thus repeating the game.

Now let us take an infant newly born,
Discuss the changes of his early dawn.
As he protests to the world with a cry,
To pink his bluish face he gives a sigh.
The soft, smooth air with its pulsatile waves
Enters the lung and fills their hidden caves;
These delicate bellows open, inflate
Their thin walled capillaries stretch, dilate,
And as the resistance within them falls,
More of the purple blood upon them calls.

Blood for the left atrium takes its leave,
And here rising pressure, as you conceive
Slams septum Primum like a swinging gate,
That's Foramen Ovale's final fate.

The midwife anxious to move to stage three,
Divides the cord and sets the infant free,
With umbilical vein empty and dry
To which Round Ligament we now apply;
And with arteries which thrombose, we're told
Each one forming and Umbilical Fold.

How then Ductus Venosus bars the way
To the flowing current of yesterday?
On this mystery fancy theories abound
But none of these I intend to expound.

Ductus Arteriorsus pulls its walls,
To a narrow tube, and lumen falls.
Though the cause of this is unknown today,
Many a physiologist will say;
It is the change in oxygen tension-

This, at least, is the present contention.

Whatever the cause of this reaction
The work of Born is now fact and sanction.
Showed that Ductus reduced to a quarter
Brings blood, reversed, to lungs from Aorta,
After some time its lining forms a heap-
A ligament, at least, in baby sheep.

Wonder then we must at least, Nature's deeds,
How well she provides for all foetal needs;
Beyond the womb she continues the care,
Prepare the infant for breathing the air!

"Science, Medicine and Poetry" was an eye-opener for me! It shows that we physicians are no less keen in showing interest and participation in literature and poetry than any other group of people outside the literary circle proper. The curious association between poetry and medicine is at least partly explained by what one writer pointed out:

"Every poet is a kind of healer, and every physician must be a kind of poet, otherwise he can not read the mysteries that lie hidden in strange organisms!"

Finally, I would like to make some comments on "Arabian Contribution to Medical Science." First, it was reassuring to read in the title "Arabian Contribution" rather than "Arabic Contribution." Many readers may think there is no difference between the two, but, in reality, there is a subtle yet huge difference. Then I was pleased to read the prologue: a quotation by Al-Kindi, the only prominent physician and writer of pure Arabic stock from that era, who said,

" It is fitting for us then not to be ashamed to acknowledge truth and to assimilate it from former generations and foreign people. For him who seeks the truth there is nothing of higher value; it never cheapens him or abases him who searches for it, but enables and honors him."

This sounded promising! Those who contributed to history and humanity should be given the credit they deserve, regardless of their ethnic or national identity. Yet, to my dismay, the article fell short in many aspects. Like many other scholars, George fell into the mistake of discrediting the pillars of Arabian medicine, the non-Arabs, and gave all the credit to the students rather than the masters (although many of the students eventually managed to become masters in their own right). Even when the non-Arab pioneers were mentioned, they were called "Arabs."

In a prefatory note to his book, *Arabian Medicine and Its Influence on the Middle Ages*, Dr. Donald Campbell says:

"The term Arabian does not necessarily imply an Arab, for the Persians and Nestorians (Assyrians) in the East, and the Spaniards and Jews in the West, took the principal part in the development of medicine which was expressed in Arabic language during the dominancy of the Empire of Islam."

As we know, when the Arabs (Moslems) came out of the Arabian Peninsula and invaded the Fertile Crescent, they took over a land that nurtured cultures and civilizations thousands of years old. Thus, Arabs did not simply start from ground zero. Their lack of knowledge left them with no choice but to rely on the local professionals in running their new state—a fact that many Arab and western scholars tend to forget by the practice of selective ignorance. Almost all of the ancient academies were established and staffed by non-Arabs. The school of Jundi-Shapur in Persia was the only center for teaching medicine in the entire Middle East, and it was almost completely staffed by Nestorian Assyrians. Many prominent physicians studied there who have become forgotten legends: their contributions are only mentioned in passing today, like the Masaweyh family, the Bukht-Yishu family, and Hunayn ibn Ishaq. None of these was an Arab. Even the teaching was in Syriac (Neo-Assyrian) for several centuries before it was replaced by Arabic. These giants were the pillars upon which Arabian medicine was built. They preserved the Greek science that came so near to perishing by collecting and translating it into Syriac first and only then into Arabic.

During his final year of medical school, George was fortunate to have fewer financial pressures. One day George was summoned into the Dean's office.

"Mr. Abouna, we have been so pleased with your performance that we thought we should help! We know it has been rough for you to work and study at the same time. The school has decided to fund your final year so that you do not have to work anymore!"

This was great news for George. It certainly gave him more time to spend with his family, to read a little more, and have some spare time for his scholarly activities. After fulfilling all the requirements and passing the final tests, George graduated from medical school and was awarded his MBBS degree in 1961.

Chapter 7

Postgraduate Training

Royal Victoria Infirmary and Newcastle University Hospital

Newcastle-Upon-Tyne

1961–1967

By the time George finished medical school, it was not difficult for him to figure out what sort of training he wanted to pursue. During his clinical rotations in medical school, he realized that surgery was meant for him. From the first moment that he saw a surgeon drawing his scalpel against the skin of a patient, George gaped in awe. His thoughts were confirmed during his first year of rotating internships, when he did his surgical rotation under Professor A. G. Lowdon of the Royal Victoria Infirmary[13], a time that proved to be most instrumental in shaping George's future career.

As a junior registrar (resident), George used to start his day at the bedside in his "uniform": a white jacket with pockets that bulged with quick reference-books, wound-dressing supplies, a small pin light, and a stethoscope. Early morning rounds were the prologue to his typical day, when all patients on the ward were seen and a list of scut work was generated. It almost seemed as if there was no end to any given day. The scut list grew longer and longer by the hour when his assignments were interrupted by more urgent tasks. Coffee breaks were literally nonexistent, and all meals were practically inhaled! One moment he was in the intensive care unit checking on a patient with deteriorating vital signs or evaluating a new patient in the emergency room for abdominal pain, and the next minute he was in the trauma bay taking part in treating a victim of a motor vehicle accident. Then was the worst—a long overnight call after a busy day only to be followed by another typical day without enough sleep! The only reason why any person would tolerate these miserable conditions is the tremendous amount of learning involved.

---

[13] **Royal Victoria Infirmary;**
Established in 1751.

Shortly after he started his junior year, George managed to break the psychological barrier that stood in the way of his knife as he pulled it against the skin of his first patient. The task proved to be addictive! From simple abscess drainage, he worked his way through line placement to appendectomies to hernia repair as he approached the end of his junior year. Through practice and perseverance over the next four years, George built up and tuned his skills with confidence. He was able to manage the adversity of surgical problems and to deal with the associated technical complexities as he progressed in his residency training. On the family front, it was during this period that George and Jennifer were blessed with two sons: Andrew in 1964 and Benjamin in 1966, making surgical residency even more challenging with a family of a wife and four children.

Of interest is that George was not only learning as a surgical resident—he was also teaching medical and other allied health students. He served as an instructor in anatomy for the university of Newcastle-upon-Tyne under Professor R. J. Scothorne (1962–1963), a post that enabled George to master his knowledge of surgical anatomy.

The final year of his residency was the most exciting yet the most difficult one. It is true that it gave George the opportunity to work on bigger cases such as gastroesophageal, hepatobiliary, pancreatic, and endocrine procedures, but it also imposed on him some direct responsibilities in the decision-making process and in taking care of his patients. It was a transitional period that took him from being a minion into an independent surgeon—a weaning process that all residents were expected to go through.

As a senior registrar, George felt at ease in the operating room. All of the motions suddenly seemed to unfold without effort —the fruits of prolonged training. Surgeries then made more sense than ever before as he became more facile with the physiological and pathological basis of surgical diseases. Among other things, George showed an unusual interest in organ system failure. Liver failure was the most intriguing for him and certainly the least treatable at that time. With his background in engineering, George embarked on a research endeavor that eventually culminated into the most innovative achievement in his entire career: the Abouna Chamber for liver support.

The last hurdle in George's way was the English Board of Surgery examination. After passing the examination, he became a Fellow of the Royal College of Surgeons (FRCS) in England in 1966.

Chapter 8

Surgical Fellowship

Organ Transplantation and Artificial Organs

University of Newcastle-upon-Tyne, UK

1967–1969

Because of his interest in academic surgery, and with continuous encouragement by Dr. Dennis Walder, George accepted a teaching position and joined the higher ranks at the University of Newcastle-upon-Tyne as an instructor and a fellow in surgery. This was a unique opportunity for him to satisfy his interests in finding some novel means for the treatment of organ failure.

George focused on patients with liver failure, many of whom would die from hepatic coma. He laid down a comprehensive plan that envisioned two goals for his research laboratory: mastering the technique of liver transplantation in animals first and searching for artificial means of supporting patients in hepatic coma until they were able to regenerate their own livers or as a bridge to liver transplantation. With his background in engineering, he started the first step by designing an apparatus that would be able to host animal livers. Then he went searching for the optimal means to prolong the preservation time of the isolated livers.

His first successful perfusion apparatus encompassed, among other things, an Aga roller, oxygenator and pump, heat exchanger, filter/bubble trap, reservoirs, flow meter, electric thermometer, and the chamber that hosted the liver. The apparatus was primed with the appropriate solutions under controlled temperature and pH. Initial experiments were faced with the problem of early congestion of the venous outflow from the liver, which jeopardized any possibility of prolonged preservation times. These technical difficulties were overcome by modifying the chamber in such a way that the liver was placed on a plastic sling that had the approximate configuration of the diaphragm. The plastic sling was subjected to intermittent oscillations that simulated normal respiratory movements, which proved to very helpful.

Once the apparatus was operational, further experiments were conducted to determine the optimal perfusion solutions for the isolated livers. Among his early findings was the fact that Ringer's lactate was not the optimal solution during the period of ischemia and hypothermia but rather a balanced electrolyte solution with added potassium, magnesium, sulphate, phosphate, glucose, insulin, and dextran, which had to be previously buffered and oxygenated.

Evaluating liver function after isolation was another research question that was addressed by George and his group. In a separate experiment using the same research design, they showed that bile output and oxygen consumption, both of which can easily be measured, gave a good indication of overall liver function, whereas the clearance of ammonia by itself was of little value.

These findings set the stage for George to take his research a step further by engaging in animal trials using isolated livers in his apparatus to support animals undergoing hepatic failure. Hepatic coma was surgically induced in a canine model while a baboon liver was isolated and preserved in the apparatus. The canine circulation was moved through the isolated liver for several hours via an A-V fistula created in the canine vessels. The initial results were quite astonishing! Many of the dogs in coma would wake up and survive for a prolonged time.

After these successes, he decided to take his work into clinical application. The first successful attempt was carried out on a child with acute hepatic coma caused by viral hepatitis. After several hours of cross-circulation with a baboon liver hosted in Abouna's chamber, the child woke up with an immediate improvement in the liver biochemical profile! The level of recovery was maintained for several days; however, no human liver became available, and the child went into irreversible hepatic coma that led to his death. The experience was reproduced for a total of four times in Newcastle-upon-Tyne. Two of the patients were able to regenerate their own livers and remained alive and well for several years!

In the midst of all these exciting findings, George was asked in 1968 to take a leave of absence for a year to support the University of Bristol transplantation program. It was during this year that Bristol attempted its first human liver transplant outside the United States. A young man in his twenties was brought to Bristol in a state of hepatic coma secondary to hepatocellular carcinoma. The chief of surgery asked Abouna whether the man could be supported using his chamber. In fact, the man responded to cross-circulation with baboon livers and woke up after several hours of support. He maintained his improved condition for several days, at which time a cadaveric human liver became available! George procured the liver and was getting ready to transplant the liver, given that he was the most experienced in animal liver transplantation. To his dismay, he was given a secondary role because the chief of surgery insisted to carry out the transplant himself eventhough he had no previous experience. The surgery was unsuccessful because of a technical error that led to hepatic artery thrombosis and failure of the graft during the immediate postoperative period. The patient again went into a hepatic coma. Although he was supported again with the chamber, no new liver was found in time and the patient died, thus leaving the door wide open for Sir Roy Calne of Cambridge University, who, a month later, was able to perform the first successful human liver transplantation outside the United States.

When the year was over, George went back in 1969 to Newcastle-upon-Tyne, where he continued his work. It was then when Thomas Starzl[14] was invited to Newcastle University as a visiting professor. Starzl was taken on a tour of transplant facilities and visited Abouna's laboratory. It was impressive enough for Starzl to take George aside and offer him a position as a fellow in clinical transplantation in Denver, Colorado, an offer that no wise man would let slip.

"George, you are wasting your time in here" said Starzl, "We are doing liver transplantation there and will need your chamber to help keep our patients alive while waiting for livers."

But the University of Newcastle-upon-Tyne was not willing to give George away. To encourage him to come back, they gave him another year of leave of absence during which he continued to draw his salary from them. He was promised that they would support him to start the clinical liver transplantation program in Newcastle upon his return.

---

[14] **Thomas E. Starzl, M.D., Ph.D. (1926 -)**

A pioneer transplant surgeon. MS 1950, MD, PhD 1952 (Northwestern University Medical School, Chicago). In the book *1,000 Years, 1,000 People*: Ranking the Men and Women Who Shaped the Millennium, Starzl was ranked 213 on its list of those whose contributions have significantly influenced history's progress. Dr. Starzl's autobiography, The Puzzle People: Memoirs of a Transplant Surgeon, was published by the University of Pittsburgh Press in 1992.

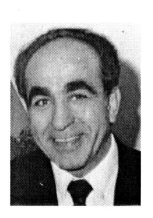

George Abouna-early years in
practice

Chapter 9
The Abouna Liver Support Apparatus
A New Extracorporeal Liver Perfusion Chamber
Newcastle-upon-Tyne
1966–1968

Necessity is the mother of all invention, and so was the invention of extracorporeal liver perfusion for the treatment of hepatic coma. The technique was developed and used simultaneously for the first time by Eiseman in the United States and by Sen in India in 1964, which was later adopted by many centers in Europe. The initial technique failed to prolong the life of isolated livers because of the serious damage to the extracorporeal liver after four to six hours of normothermic perfusion, which made them incapable of supporting life.

In his laboratory research, George adapted the existing technique and embarked on experimentation with different components of the physical environment of the isolated livers, the circuitry, and the fluids used for perfusion and preservation. He was able to design a new perfusion chamber, which, along with some changes in the circuitry and perfusion fluids used, was successful in prolonging liver preservation times after which the organs were still good for transplantation. It took more than 50 experiments on the perfusion of pig livers and another 14 experiments in which isolated and perfused pig livers were used to support calves undergoing experimental hepatic failure before the technique was taken into clinical experimentation on human subjects.

The technique was applied seven times on four human subjects in hepatic failure using isolated pig livers, with encouraging results. The experience was published, along with a detailed description of the new chamber and its application in the *Lancet* in 1968.

The chamber consists of three components: the outer container, the liver diaphragm, and the lid. The outer container is a stainless-steel cylinder 10 inches in diameter and 6 inches high. Around its open top is welded a flange 2 inches in diameter and 1 inch high that has eight equally spaced slots to receive corresponding studs from the metal ring of the liver diaphragm. On one side of the container, near its base, are two ports one-half and one-quarter inch in diameter for the passage of the inferior vena cava tubing and the "ascetic fluid" tubing of the liver diaphragm, respectively. On the opposite side is another port seven-eighths inch in diameter that accepts standard anesthesia tubing and connects the external container to a ventilator.

Mounted on the sides of the outer container are brackets for holding a small stainless-steel heat exchanger, a bile reservoir, and an expandable manometer scale. The container stands on three telescopic legs. It can be sterilized by autoclaving.

The liver diaphragm is made of soft polyvinyl chloride and has the approximate configuration of a normal diaphragm. The diaphragm is suspended by a stainless-steel ring that is sandwiched between two layers of the same material. From the lower surface of the ring project eight studs through slots in the flange of the outer container. To the concave bottom of the liver diaphragm are welded two plastic tubes, each 6 inches in length; the larger one, for the passage of the vena cava cannula, is one-half inch in diameter, and the smaller one, for the drainage of the "ascetic fluid," is one-quarter inch in diameter. The liver diaphragm, which is disposable, is constructed of siliconized, prepacked, sterilized ethylene oxide.

The lid is an open stainless-steel cylinder 14 and one-quarter inches in diameter and 2 and one-half inches high, with an observation window 7 and one-half inches in diameter. It fits snugly over the top of the outer container. On its upper surface are two slots of one-quarter inch diameter for the passage of the portal vein and the hepatic artery cannulae from the liver. At its side are two other slots for the passage of the bile duct cannula and the thermometer cable. Over the top of the lid, covering the observation window is placed a tight-fitting transparent plastic hood with two holes that correspond to the portal and hepatic artery cannulae. When the lid is in position, the liver inside the chamber is thus completely sealed from the atmosphere.

The modifications mimicked, as closely as possible, the physiological environment of the liver in vivo. The liver diaphragm and the oscillatory movements help to maintain even perfusion by regularly filling and emptying the liver sinusoids. During every positive pressure cycle, the hepatic venous pressure oscillates by two to three cm of water in a manner not unlike that in the normal animal. Of interest, the liver maintains its color, consistency, and functions for more than 10 hours of hypothermic perfusion. Other advantages include most parts in contact with animal liver and patient's blood being disposable; during perfusion, the chamber is completely sealed, thus maintaining sterility and humidity; the circuit is a closed system that requires as little as 500 ml of blood for priming; the design allows high-flow perfusion without causing hypotension; and safety has been optimized by placing automatic warning systems to guard against air embolism or exsanguinations. Since then, the system has been adjusted several times and thus can be used for prolonged hypothermic preservation of livers intended for transplantation. This innovative work was published in several issues of the Lancet and the British Journal of Surgery.

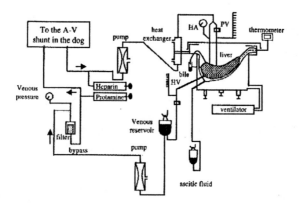

Schematic drawing of the Abouna Liver Support
Apparatus

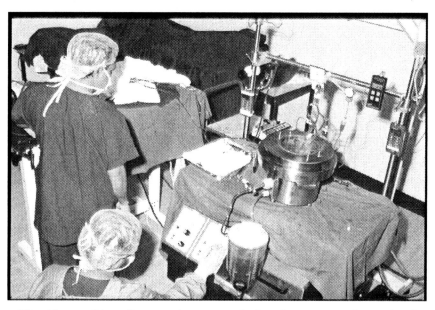

The Abouna Liver Support Apparatus during the support of an animal with hepatic failure.

Chapter 10
Clinical Organ Transplantation Fellowship
Universities of Colorado and Medical College of Virginia
Denver, Colorado, and Richmond, Virginia, USA
1969–1971

It was a great opportunity for George to start his clinical transplant training under Starzl, the first person in the world to perform a successful liver transplantation in a human subject. He packed his chamber, along with his research ideas, and headed to Denver. George also had an excellent opportunity to exchange expertise with other surgeons under Starzl. Israel Penn was among the closest to him[15].

In Denver, George was able to apply his perfusion chamber on three or four patients successfully. One such experience was dramatic enough to be published in the *Lancet*. Many lessons were learned from that case, most of which were innovative and much needed.

In summary, a 23-year-old man undergoing hepatic coma secondary to hepatitis was flown while on mechanical ventilator to Denver from New Mexico for possible liver transplantation. After evaluation, he was placed on extracorporeal hepatic support using pig livers around midnight on April 14th, 1970. The patient showed progressive improvement that enabled him to go off the ventilator. By the fourth liver perfusion, he regained full consciousness and was able to give an account of his earlier illness and had some food. Eight days later, he deteriorated to the point that he was put back on the extracorporeal perfusion system using pig liver. However, 40 minutes into the procedure, it was stopped because the patient went into anaphylactic shock. This led to the use of different animal species such as baboon, monkey, calf, and even a cadaveric human liver. With 12 hepatic perfusions, along with some exchange transfusions

---

[15] **Israel Penn (1930 -)**
A pioneer in transplantation surgery. Penn was born in Lithuania, graduated from Witwatersrand Medical School in South Africa, and became a fellow of the Royal college of Surgeons of England in 1956. He later immigrated to USA where he reached his pinnacle of success.

to correct coagulopathies, the patient was brought out of hepatic coma several times in the hope that the center could find a suitable human liver for transplantation. Six weeks after admission, the patient required hemodialysis for renal failure. However dialysis-induced hypotension, in addition to electrolyte imbalance, soon pushed the patient into a new coma.

Hopes were revived the next day, when a cadaveric liver became available: a rare opportunity back then. Everybody was happy for the patient because that would have been his only chance for a meaningful survival. The liver was not transplanted because Starzl was in the hospital recuperating from an operation for a prolapsed disc and could not lead the team! Because of that, Israel Penn asked George to approach Starzl and ask his permission to go head with the transplant without him instead of losing such a precious organ. To their dismay, Starzl did not give his blessing! Being the pioneer and the most experienced surgeon, he thought he should be the one to lead the team. Starzl told George, "You remember I told you that what you are doing is a Nobel Prize work, and I as the chief of transplantation should be the one to do the transplant for this patient". Instead, he suggested placing the human liver in Abouna's chamber to help bring the patient out of his most recent coma. Hopefully another liver would become available.

Both George and Israel had no say in the matter. They did what they were asked to do. The human liver functioned in the chamber for 35 hours with no complications or any evidence for rejection! During this perfusion, the patient regained full consciousness and recommenced normal eating. Four days, later the patient went into coma again after hypotension caused by dialysis and gastrointestinal bleeding. The patient was put again on the extracorporeal liver perfusion. The first pig liver was rejected within three hours. A second pig liver was successfully used for more than six hours under heavy steroid coverage, after which spontaneous breathing and full consciousness were restored. The patient was able to eat for four more days before his conditions deteriorated again. Within two more days, he was back on the perfusion machine using a baboon liver. After 22 hours of perfusion, spontaneous breathing and consciousness were regained for the eighth time since admission. However, so far, the patient had shown no evidence of spontaneous liver regeneration. Four days later, he went into coma again, but this time he could not be supported by extracorporeal perfusion because of vasomotor instability caused by gram-negative sepsis. He died after battling hepatic and renal failure for 76 days, a record survival time for a man in his condition. The battle was supported by a series of 16 extracorporeal liver perfusions from 10 pigs, 3 baboons, 1 calf, 1 monkey, and 1 human, supplemented by 20 exchange transfusions. This exceptional case was published in the Lancet in 1971.

Many lessons were learned from this unique experience—extracorporeal liver perfusion could restore consciousness and spontaneous breathing; the livers used could clear bilirubin and were able to synthesize factors II, V, and IX; perfusion with pig liver led to sensitization, in contrast to baboon liver; and no antibodies were formed against human cells.

Today and after more than three decades, we can still question the way Starzl had handled the situation. Was it ethical for Starzl to deny a desperate patient an operation that could have saved his life? Was it justified for Starzl to block the surgery because he could not operate? Was he really acting in the best interest of the patient, or was he after his own glory and ego?

Certainly, these may sound controversial questions with no clear answers. But it was no surprise that, more than three decades later George, when presented this case as an example of the applications of his chamber during a national transplant meeting, Starzl approached him and acknowledged that it was a mistake on his part to not allow the transplant to proceed without him.

On the clinical side, both George and Israel reported their experience with the psychological disturbances associated with organ transplantation. Data collected from 292 renal and 36 hepatic recipients showed a high incidence of postoperative psychiatric problems, most of which were reactive in nature and responded to a friendly milieu, such as the avoidance of isolation techniques and the availability of psychotherapeutic support groups.

Impressed with his pioneering work in liver perfusion, David Hume[16], a chairman and professor of surgery at the Medical College of Virginia, offered George a faculty position as an assistant professor of surgery. He provided George with every possible help to establish a new research laboratory in preparation for a program in liver transplantation. In addition to his clinical duties, George found more opportunities to use his chamber. In 1972, he reported in the *British Medical Journal* on two young patients who were brought out of their hepatic coma after 13 and one-half and 16

---

[16] **David Milford Hume (1917-1973)**
Stuart McGuire Professor of Surgery at the Medical College of Virginia. A pioneer in transplantation surgery who is credited for developing a simpler technique for renal transplantation involving placement of the graft kidney in the iliac fossa, obviating the need for removal of the non-functioning organ. He died by crashing his small plain in California.

and one-half hours of liver perfusion using baboon livers. Debra Jackson, age 13, and Yvonne Royster, age 24, were both the victims of fulminating viral hepatitis who were only hours away from death if had not been for George's intervention. Both patients turned out to be long-term survivors after regenerating their own livers, and they led normal lives thereafter. The incredible recovery of both patients made it to the national news in February 7th, 1972, when *Time* magazine reported the story of both patients and commended the method because it did not involve long waits or inordinate costs. Admittedly, it is only a bridge until the native liver recovers or is replaced by a transplant.

Chapter 11
Medical College of Georgia
Augusta, Georgia
1971–1973

After completing his work with David Hume in Virginia, George was supposed to return to University of Newcastle-upon- Tyne, but he could not turn down the many offers he received in the United States. He finally took a position as a consultant surgeon at the Medical College of Georgia. He expanded the already existing small transplant unit, which was mostly engaged in renal transplantation for the eastern and southern parts of Georgia. At the same time, George continued his work on liver support techniques and was planning to establish a clinical liver transplantation program.

George's fame had preceded him to Georgia. It was there when one day that he received a phone call from Jimmy Carter[17], the governor of Georgia, asking him whether he could take care of a friend's wife. Apparently, she had hepatorenal syndrome in Pensacola, Florida when she was flown to Augusta on a ventilator. She was the first patient successfully treated by simultaneous hemodialysis and liver hemoperfusion for liver failure and hepatorenal syndrome. She woke up for several days until she lost her airway by accidental disconnection from the ventilator. The resultant hypoxia pushed her back into an irreversible hepatic coma, and she eventually died. This unique case was published in the journal of Surgery in 1973.

The repeated success stories put George under the spotlight. After he arrived in Augusta, many patients were referred to the Medical College of Georgia under his care. It was then when Jimmy Carter wrote a letter to the director of the National Institute of Health in support of securing

---

[17] **James Earl Carter, Jr. (1924 -)**
The 39th President of the United States was born and raised in a farming family in Georgia. In 1946 he graduated form the Naval Academy in Annapolis, Maryland. After several years in politics, he was elected the Governor of Georgia in 1970, then the president of the United States in 1976 for one term. In 2002, Carter was awarded the Nobel Peace Prize for his decades of untiring effort to find peaceful solutions to international conflicts, to advance democracy and human rights, and to promote economic and social development.

some grants for further research on liver failure treatment alternatives. As indicated below, this letter shows the strong commitment and support by the governor for a liver transplantation program.

September 29, 1972
Dr. Robert G. Marston
Director
National Institute of Health
9000 Rockville Pike
Bethesda, Maryland
Dear Dr. Marston:

I am deeply concerned about a grant request from the Medical College of Georgia, which has been submitted, to the National Institute of Health for liver transplant work.

We are very fortunate in Georgia to have brought to our Medical School, Dr. George Abouna, from England, whose work has brought new hope for many victims of liver failure.

I have been following up with the kidney transplant and dialysis program since I have been Governor and have become interested in the research going on at the Medical College of Georgia in the liver transplant work. We have patients coming from distant parts of the country to the Medical College to seek help with liver ailments due to Dr. Abouna's presence there. The President of the Medical College who was former Chairman of The Department of Surgery is personally interested in this project. Dr. Abouna has told me that in resubmitting this request, he has made every effort to conform to the suggestions, which were given him by the NIH last year. If I can be of any assistance in expediting this grant request, please let me know. I feel very strongly that this liver research directly affects the lives of many Georgians as well as many Americans.

With best wishes,
Sincerely,

Jimmy Carter
JC/llj

Despite all the efforts, adequate funds could not be secured. In addition, many logistic problems stood in the way of such a program. During this time, George was contacted by Sir Michael Woodruff[18] of the Edinburgh Royal Infirmary[19], who asked George to join him there, as he was planning to retire in a couple of years. Sir Michael Woodruff viewed George to be his perfect successor to lead the Nuffield transplant unit. George was also contacted by Dr. McPhedran of the University of Calgary inviting him to head the transplant program in Calgary, Alberta, Canada.

---

[18] **Prof Sir Michael (Francis Addison) Woodruff (1911-2001);**
MB, BS (Melbourne) 1937, MD 1940, MS 1941; FRCS 1946 (England). He was knighted in 1969 for his contributions to medicine.
[19] **Royal Infirmary of Edinburgh;**
Established in 1870.

Chapter 12
Edinburgh Royal Infirmary, University of Edinburgh
Edinburgh, Scotland, UK
1973–1974

After four years of clinical transplantation experience in the United States, George felt that it was time for him and his family to return to the country that he considered his second home. The position offered by Sir Woodruff carried great potential for a successful career in academic surgery. He was certainly hoping that he could start a liver transplantation program in Edinburgh.

While he was engaged in clinical transplantation at the Nuffield transplant unit, George was fortunate to become among the pioneers in the history of transplantation in the United Kingdom. He is credited for successfully performing the first living-donor kidney transplantation in the United Kingdom. Before that, all transplants were cadaveric in origin, because living organ donation was not permitted. But the expanding need for organs put substantial pressure on the powers that be to allow such a venue. Shortly thereafter, he was successful in performing the first renal transplant for a pediatric patient in the United Kingdom.

To his dismay, George's vision for his future in Edinburgh was clouded by a family storm. His eldest daughter, Linda, wanted to go back to North America. She had gotten so used to living in the United States that she could not accustom herself to living in Edinburgh. Against her family's will, she packed her belonging and flew back to Augusta, Georgia. Out of concern for her teenager daughter, Jennifer had no choice but to take her other three children and pack back to Georgia until a solution could be found.

This was a tremendous pressure on George that he could not hide. He explained his situation to Sir Michael Woodruff. During his last few days in Edinburgh, George was the guest of Sir Michael and Mrs. Woodruff at their residence, during which Sir Michael Woodruff told George that he was sad to see him leave but that he was right to put his family above all else. "Your family should come first," Sir Michael Woodruff told him. "If you are not happy at home, you cannot be happy at work." With these words in mind, George accepted reality and started to pack to go back to North America.

Chapter 13

Faculty of Medicine, University of Calgary

Calgary, Alberta, Canada

1974–1975

When he was forced to return to North America, George reconsidered an earlier offer to join the Faculty of Medicine at the University of Calgary. He became a member of the preexisting renal transplant team and the head of the newly established multidisciplinary organ transplant program. This was a good compromise for his family to reunite and live under one roof.

After arrival at Foothills hospital (the medical center for the faculty of medicine), George had to make some changes in the way things were run to be able to expand their services and cope with the increasing demand for renal transplantation. These changes were initially met with some unhappiness on the part of the nursing staff, who complained of a lack of communication between them and the leader of the team. George was understanding and worked on resolving the issues. In due time, the renal transplant unit worked in harmony and tripled the number of cases treated within a short period of time. This was also matched with a significant decrease in postoperative morbidity, from 40% down to only 5%.

On July 30th, 1975, Foothills hospital had its first experience with a human liver transplantation, which proved to be a unique one by several accounts. In addition to its being George's first case, it was also the first liver transplant to be completed successfully in western Canada, the first in the world performed on a patient with ileostomy, the first performed for cholangiocarcinoma secondary to ulcerative colitis, and the first in which the liver was taken from a child (16 years old) and transplanted into an adult. After 16 years of having ulcerative colitis, Rob MacKenzie underwent total abdominal proctocolectomy and a permanent ileostomy. Several years later, he developed progressive jaundice and was referred to Foothills hospital for further treatment. He was found to have a nonresectable tumor of the liver for which a draining procedure was performed while he waited for a liver donor.

The operation itself was challenging because of technical difficulties caused by duplicated hepatic artery of the donor liver and the mismatch in size between the donor and recipient vessels. To complicate matters, the patient went into cardiac arrest during the anhepatic phase. CPR was started while George was performing the vascular anastomoses. After

40 minutes of CPR, the patient was revived, and the graft showed good function, as depicted by immediate production of bile. The surgery lasted 10 hours. When Rob left the hospital several weeks later, he told a reporter from *The Albertan* that he "felt real good."

However, MacKenzie's good health did not last very long: 7 and one-half months later, he complained of abdominal and back pain. An examination revealed the presence of bone metastases. Chemotherapy was not effective, and the patient died some 9 months after the transplant. This historic accomplishment was published in the Canadian Medical Journal in 1977.

Chapter 14
The Calgary Incident: A Controversy or a Conspiracy?
Calgary, Alberta, Canada
1975–1978

After only a year of unprecedented success in renal transplantation at Foothills Hospital in Calgary, George was caught off guard on June 15th, 1975, by a baseless suspension from the renal transplant team, followed by withdrawal of his privileges for the procedure without notice. From George's perspective, it all stemmed back to the fact that, when he joined the transplant unit at the University of Calgary, it was small and inefficient, performing only a handful of kidney transplants a year. The outcome was modest at best, with a high morbidity rate. George had imposed many changes that were overdue if the unit was to excel. Although those changes were welcomed by many, they created much animosity among a few others.

Soon after his arrival at Foothills hospital, George rolled up his sleeves and launched a program that enabled the unit to triple its renal transplants and performed the first successful liver transplant in Western Canada in less than a year! The transplant morbidity rate was reduced 5% from the 40% rate before his arrival. As might be expected, there was a conflict of interest, and George was soon considered to be a serious professional threat by his transplant partner, who was already well established in Calgary. The tension escalated to the point that kidney transplantation was suspended at Foothills Hospital on May 30th, 1975.

Apparently, Dr. N. T. McPhedran[20], Professor and Head of the Division of Surgery at the Faculty of Medicine, University of Calgary, recommended the suspension and withdrawal of George's privileges. To make a plausible case, renal transplant statistics were falsified before the hospital board to show that George's results were inferior to those of his partner, and he indeed managed to persuade the hospital board to accept

---

[20] **N. T. McPhedran, MD (1924 -);**
The former Head of Surgery at the Faculty of Medicine, University of Calgary. He moved from Toronto to Calgary in 1969 to establish an academic surgery department at the faculty of medicicne. He stepped down in 1984 and currently holds the title of "Professor Emeritus".

these fraudulent allegations. To make matters worse, the hospital issued a press release alleging that the transplant work of Dr. Abouna was below expectations.

Acting in self-defense, George requested an appeal before the hospital board, but his appeal, which was initially scheduled in June and then delayed to September, was stalled! The matter did not remain a secret for long. Patients and their advocates started to wonder what was happening behind the closed doors. After failing to unravel the truth and to obtain justice internally, George was forced to take the matter to the courts. The incident created more controversy and media attention than any previous medical or health-related issue in Calgary. In due time, Calgary, its university, and its government were thrust into the national spotlight.

On July 17th, 1975, Fred Haeseker, a staff writer for the *Calgary Herald*, reported on the first public reaction to the matter under the title, "Abouna appeal stalled—Patients petition government." Patients of Dr. George Abouna formed a committee of 25 patients, chaired by Pat Moncrieff of Lethbridge, who had undergone a renal transplant surgery performed by Dr. Abouna a few months earlier. The committee collected more than 500 signatures on a petition to be presented to Mr. Gordon Miniely, Alberta Hospitals Minister, imploring him to investigate the Foothills renal and transplant units. The committee accused the Foothills hospital administration of stalling Dr. Abouna's appeal and playing with human lives by stopping transplant surgery, citing the recent death of a patient waiting for a kidney transplant. In a separate incident, two donor kidneys that became available were wasted for the same reason. Many patients interviewed by Mr. Haeseker had recently moved their care to Dr. Abouna because they wanted the best for themselves. In the midst of this ordeal, they all wondered what could be more important than the fate of the patients.

---

[21] **The honorable Ralph Klein (1942 -);**
Mr. Klein was elected leader of the Progressive Conservative Party in 1992, the same year he was sworn in as Alberta's 12th Premier until the present day. He is credited for revamping and opening up the government's decision-making process, balancing the budget, and paying down the debt. In 1980 he was elected Calgary's 32nd Mayor, a post he won for three terms. Mr. Klein's major accomplishments include the 1988 Olympic Winter Games, Calgary's Light Rail Transit System and protection of the Bow River. In 1989 he was appointed Minister of Environment through which he oversaw the development of the Alberta Environmental Protection and Enhancement Act. Mr. Klein has received numerous honors and awards for his outstanding achievements in Alberta.

Dr. Abouna's patients took the matter a step further by meeting Mr. Ralph Klein[21], the Senior Civic Affairs reporter with CFCN Television and Radio. They wanted the public to hear what they had to say about the man who cared for them and was always responsive to their needs; a man who was being drummed out for no reason other than professional jealousy. To investigate the matter, Mr. Klein tracked down Dr. Abouna and conducted an interview with him but could not hear the perspective of those in the opposite camp. Dr. McPhedran and the other renal unit physicians were very reluctant to come forward and talk about what they had against Dr. Abouna. Finally, Mr. Klein reported on what he was able to gather. In response, the Foothills' hospital held a press release to contradict Mr. Klein's report.

But what about the position of the nursing staff in the renal transplant unit? On October 1st, 1975, Paul Legall, a staff writer for the *Albertan,* reported on the matter under the title, "Nurses side with Abouna." In a letter sent by the nursing staff to G. Balck, chairman of the hospital board of management, the nurses spoke very highly of Dr. Abouna and hoped that the hospital would allow him to continue his work. Although the nurses admitted that the changes made by Dr. Abouna created some unhappiness and misunderstanding, they acknowledged that, given his high expectations, Dr. Abouna had responded favorably and that the differences had been resolved to the point that the transplant team was working together smoothly and in harmony.

But the conflict of interest was too deep for such appeals to be effective. The perpetrators entrenched themselves and were ready to push with their allegations to the end. Even under the public and the media pressures, the government of Alberta refused to intervene! The official statement was that the government did not want to jeopardize hospitals' autonomy! As for George, no words were enough to describe his feelings. He had lost his job and his privileges to operate; his reputation was battered, and his career appeared to be ruined. In June 1976, the University of Calgary allowed his appointment as an Associate Professor of Surgery at the medical school to lapse. Facing a financial disaster as the sole caretaker of his family of a wife and four teenaged children, George had no choice but to accept a favor from a fellow physician, who offered him a job in his medical office, to be able to survive.

It was not until March 1977 that the case was argued in a three-day trial before Mr. MacDonald, Alberta Supreme Court Justice. Many facts about the plot had surfaced during the period preceding the trial. Professor McPhedran, the head of the Division of Surgery, tried to rectify the matter by circulating an apology to all members of the Division of Surgery several months before the scheduled court date. Three months after the trial, Justice MacDonald released a 34-page judgment in favor of Dr. Abouna.

On June 9th, 1977, Gordon Lee, a staff writer for the *Albertan,* reported the details of the judgment under the title, "Abouna awarded $100,000 in suit against hospital." The judge had found that the hospital board had violated the "rule of natural justice" by suspending Abouna's hospital staff privileges without notice and without giving Abouna a chance to be heard, in effect cutting off his life's blood. Perhaps more important was the fact that the court found the data provided by the perpetrators to be obviously wrong. Justice MacDonald found the hospital guilty of wrongful dismissal, and proper remedy for wrong dismissal, he affirmed, was an award of damages. Dr. Abouna was also awarded the costs of the lawsuit. Justice MacDonald concluded his judgment by stating that the result of the unfortunate events of that period was to hurt Dr. Abouna's reputation, which was held in "high regard" elsewhere in North America before the Foothills controversy.

The court judgment was big relief for the Abouna family after two long years of stress. This victory of truth was enough for George to forget the past and look toward the future. He agreed to settle, out of court in return for a written public apology and payment of token damages, a separate legal action of defamation against Dr. McPhedran, because he did not wish to subject a fellow physician to the damaging ordeal of a public trial.

On June 11th, 1977, Gordon Lee reported in the *Albertan* the details of the settlement. The announcement was made through a brief press release issued through the offices of Code Hunter, a city law firm, and signed by Abouna and McPhedran.

In his letter dated June 10th, 1977, and on the letterhead of the University of Calgary, Faculty of Medicine, Division of Surgery, Dr. McPhedran wrote:

"I am writing to you for the purpose of withdrawing the comments that were made by me at the monthly meetings of the Division of Surgery at Foothills Hospital on November 3, 1975 and December 1, 1975 in respect of yourself and the use of research data that has been allegedly obtained from Dr. Gordon Dixon of the Division of Medical Biochemistry in this faculty. The comments which I made at those meetings with respect to the use of such research data by you were based on information that had been supplied to me by Dr. R.B. Church which, at that time, I believed was true. Since then I have inquired into this matter, and I am now convinced that the information upon which my statements were based was not correct."

"I wish to apologize for this error on my part and any damage to your professional reputation and standing which such statements may have caused. I wish to add that I personally regard you as having integrity as a research scientist, and as a competent academic surgeon."

"As part of our settlement and in a further attempt to minimize any damage to your career and reputation, I have written to Dr. Le Riche of the College of Physicians and Surgeons of Alberta and to Dr. Graham of the Royal College of Physicians and Surgeons of Canada asking them not to pursue the complaints about you that were made by me on September 30, 1975....".

The news was not only exciting for George but also for those who believed in his cause. In a private letter sent to Dr. Abouna on June 16th, 1977, Mr. Rod Sykes[22], the Mayor of Calgary, wrote," I have just finished reading a copy of the judgment, and I am shocked at the finding of the judge that the charts and statistics presented were fabricated to produce a result other than the truth. It seems to me that, on the basis of such a finding, the minister of health must take some action in connection with the Hospital Board and with those members of the Medical Advisory Committee involved. After all there is very little difference between the murder of a man and the deliberate destruction of everything he represents and everything his family has."

"I was convinced from the beginning of the justice of your position, and I was appalled at the refusal to give you a fair hearing and, indeed, the apparent obstruction put in your way at every level of administration and government right up to the Provincial Cabinet. Indeed, one Cabinet Minister who would have supported you told me that he had been advised to keep out of the matter by the Premier's Office, and others had a similar experience."

"I don't suppose that anyone can understand what you and your family have suffered in this past two years but you have my most sincere admiration for your courage in the face of every adversity and injustice that could be put in your way; and, certainly, the community is better for you having fought your battle and won. It is not in the nature of affairs that you will ever be adequately compensated, and most of your satisfaction must come from knowing that you did what had to be done and that those people who tried to destroy you may think twice before they try again with anyone else."

[22] **James Rodney (Rod) W. Sykes (1929 -);**
In 1969, Mr. Sykes ran for the office of the Mayor in Calgary and was elected with the biggest majority in the history of the city at that time. He served three terms before resigning prior to the 1977 election. Since then he has continued his activities in property development and, in addition, writes a regular column for the Calgary Sun newspaper.

Mr. Sykes concluded his letter by saying,

"I wish you and your family the greatest happiness and success in the future. I do hope that you will not remember Calgary solely in the light of your sad experience but rather in the light of your triumph which is a triumph of justice."

But the triumph did not return matters to business as usual. The judgment did not ensure the reinstatement of Dr. Abouna to his hospital privileges at Foothills Hospital, and the case was far from over. The public was becoming as frustrated as George in managing this ordeal and had lost faith in its health care system. The letter sent by Mr. Sykes, the Mayor of Calgary, to Gordon Miniely, the Minister of Hospitals and Medical Care, about the Abouna affair is a reflection of such frustration. In his letter dated August 3rd, 1977, Mr. Sykes wrote," I attach a copy of an editorial taken from the *Albertan* of July 29th, 1975. Your reported position then you would not interfere with the Abouna case barring incompetence or impropriety on the part of the Hospital Board. The editorial goes on to say that the hospital exists to serve the public and that it is your responsibility to see that it puts that duty first."

"I have no doubt that you have read the judgment of Mr. Justice MacDonald in this matter, and it is impossible, on the basis of that judgment, to come to any conclusion other than that the hospital did not put the welfare of the public first and that the Board did act improperly— to put it mildly!"

"It seems to me that the MacDonald judgment clearly places the responsibility for acting on your shoulders, and I would like to know why Dr. Abouna has not been fully reinstated in all his hospital privileges."

Mr. Sykes concluded his latter by saying, "While I did not agree with your original decision not to intervene, perhaps because I thought I knew more about the matter than was generally known, I did respect your right to take the position you did. However, events have proven that your position was not the correct one and your commitment must surely be to act to see that justice is done, both to Dr. Abouna and to the people of this city. Accordingly, I do hope that you will take this request seriously and not dismiss it as merely another political contribution to an unhappy affair. The judgment makes it clear where the political contributions came from, and your responsibility in this matter now requires to be dealt with finally."

On a larger scale, the *Albertan* published an opinion titled, "Operate!" on March 6th, 1978, which stated:

"Albertans—and Dr. George Abouna—deserve a diagnosis and a prescribed remedy for the pallor which must lie over this province's medical community as a result of Dr. Abouna's 2 and a one- half year-long struggle against his wrongful dismissal from Foothills Hospital."

"Whatever the proper method of diagnosis is, a provincial judicial inquiry, as Social Credit Party Leader Bob Clark suggested last week, is not clear. But, what is becoming clear in the wake of Alberta Supreme Court's finding (upheld by the Appeals Court) is that the Foothills Hospital's Board of managers acted improperly in dismissing transplant specialist Dr. Abouna, and that this province's reputation in the international medical community has been tarnished. In such a situation, the provincial government must see the need for some action on its part to clear the air. It can no longer hide behind an insistence on hospital's autonomy, as it has done throughout the long Abouna case."

"The diagnosis and cure should obviously be applied to the cause of the province's image problems in the medical community. Hospital boards must be seen to be discharging their authority- regarding allowing doctors' hospital rights and other matters—in a responsible and accountable way."

"In November, 1975, we said 'the Abouna file is proving hard to close,' and suggested some preventive medicine so the career-harming, confidence-shattering incident might not repeat itself: an independent tribunal to which appeals of staff-privileges decisions of the hospital boards might be taken. The Abouna file is still not closed in 1978, and the province should perform some immediate and curative 'doctoring'."

In spite of the tremendous public pressure exercised in this case, *bureaucracy* proved again to be stronger than the laws of natural justice. Dr. Abouna realized that his career as a transplant surgeon in Calgary was beyond salvage. To complicate matters even more, an escalation of tensions at home culminated in a divorce that sent George and his wife Jennifer on their separate ways. Finally, George accepted a position as a Professor and Chairman of the newly established department of Surgery at the Faculty of Medicine, University of Kuwait. The new appointment seemed to be an answer to his prayers: to break him out of the state of inertia that he had lived in for almost two years and to open a new door to the future.

It is interesting to know that even after George had left for Kuwait, the battle was not over, and the knights of justice refused to drop their swords!

One such knight was Mr. Roy Farran[23], the Solicitor General for the Government of Alberta in 1975. In his article in the *Albertan* in 1980, titled, "Taking a stand," he wrote, "What the hell do you stand for, Farran? This is a question that has been put to me in different ways more than once."

Mr. Farran goes on to describe his stance in the Abouna's case:

"Of course, if I believe in a mobile society, I believe that the bigger they are the harder they'll fall. So I have more empathy with small business than with large corporations and I say what I think."

"To give you an example, I will cite the case of Dr. Abouna, the brilliant transplant surgeon in Calgary. His shafting by the establishment made me more ashamed than anything that has ever happened in public life."

"He was a perfectionist with whom lesser people found it difficult to work. Because he received a salary from the university as opposed to the normal medical fee-for-service, he could spend more time in the hospital. And he made the mistake of criticizing his colleagues. The establishment closed ranks and booted him all the way to Kuwait while the government stood by like Pontius Pilate, washing its hands. Because I didn't say what I thought loud enough, I've had it on my conscience ever since."

Along the same lines, many faculty colleagues of Dr. Abouna requested that the Canadian Association of University Teachers (CAUT)[24] conduct an independent investigation in the handling of the Abouna case. Accordingly, the CAUT governing council, at its meeting in Ottawa on May 15th, 1980, voted to place the Board of Governors of the University of Calgary under the third stage of censure, under which CAUT recommends that faculty members not accept appointments at the university. The standoff escalated when the President of the University of Calgary, Dr. Norman Wagner, took no action to resolve the standoff. The CAUT council voted during its meeting in Ottawa on May 13th, 1982, to impose the third stage of

---

[23] **Roy Alexander Farran (1921 -);**
A professional soldier, newspaper publisher, novelist, Alderman and Member of the Legislative Assembly of Alberta, was born in England. Arriving in Calgary, Alberta, in the mid 1950's he was employed by the Calgary Herald and subsequently established the North Hill News as publisher and owner. Between 1961-1963 and 1964-1971, Mr. Farran served as Alderman for Calgary. He then served with the Provincial Government as an MLA for the constituency of Calgary North and as Minister of Telephones and Utilities and later Solicitor General (1975). Mr. Farran retired from Government service in 1978.

[24] **CAUT;**
The Canadian Association of University Teachers.

censure on the office of the President of the University of Calgary, which had already been in effect on the Board of Governors of the University since 1980.

In 1989 the censure was still in effect. The CAUT council contacted Dr. Abouna to start some channels of communication with the University of Calgary. The council made it clear that it was willing to carry the censure as long as it took until justice was served. But Dr. Abouna asked the council to lift the censure! "It is time to forgive and forget," he said. Even now, and after almost three decades, Dr. McPhedran continues to defend his decision! In a telephone interview he said it was hard to work with Dr. Abouna yet he offered nothing to support his stance.

Although Abouna's case has rested between the folds of the past, the fruits of his work in Calgary have not. During the ordeal, George was consoled by the flashing words of his patient, Pat Moncrieff:

Abouna!!
He walked into the hospital
His position obvious ...
To keep his oath, and to do his job
Of taking care of the sick.

He thought his colleagues would do the same
Took him awhile to realize ...
They played a different game.

He did not drive a flashy car
Nor care for jet-set parties
His work came first you see
And so the trouble started.

He thought his job was to do the best
In what he chose to do
To get these people well again – Put
back at jobs and school.

He was a stranger in this land
His skin a little dark
But the brilliance of this man
was soon to leave a mark.

And so they got together,

Said "This man has got to go"
We'll tell a story so good
No one will ever know.
We'll stick together no matter what
And soon this man will be forgot.

But these fine people forgot one thing
His patients who loved him will never forget him.

We know the sorrow that he boar
The road he walked alone
May God have mercy on their souls
And their hearts of stone.

His head is bowed and his heart is broke
But he does not walk alone
The man with scarred hands and feet
Who walked that same road too
Walks down that long road with him – whispering:
"Forgive them they know not what they do."

Today, George remembers Calgary solely in the light of his positive experience there; an experience that is still cherished by those who lived to talk about it. In a telephone interview with the honorable Ralph Klein, the Premier of Alberta, he remembers the positive impact George left on his patients who did everything they could to support him through his ordeal, of whom many led normal lives. One such patient, Karen McKinnon, celebrated in 1999 her 25 years of success after she received a kidney from her sister, Linda Neufield. Karen told Howard May, a reporter for the *Calgary Herald,* that Dr. Abouna's surgery not only gave her normal life but also helped her to develop a fierce sense of independence. A single mother of two, she refused to accept welfare. She went back to school, got her degree and started to teach art at James Fowler High School in Calgary. Even after Karen's death 3 years later, her daughter Sabrina delBen found some comfort in writing to Dr. Abouna. On March 23rd, 2003 she wrote, "It is with regrets I write to tell you of my mother's passing. I wanted to let you know just what an impact you made on our lives. Not only did you perform a life saving transplant, but you gave mom the motivation to survive. She named her "new" kidney "George"- and George was the only healthy, cancer free part of her when she died. I know you helped many people in your medical career- but to me- you gave me 28 more years with a mother! I can not begin to tell you how much that has meant to me and my brother, Colin." Sabrina concluded her letter saying, "Hope is an art - continue to practice it".

Stories like Karen's not only give those waiting in line for their transplantation a real hope but also give surgeons like George the power and the will to carry on with their mission. "If it is all up to me now," Mr. Ralph Klein says, "I would like to see Dr. Abouna back in Alberta". Mr. Klein had recently met with Dr. Abouna in Calgary exploring possible venues for Abouna's return.

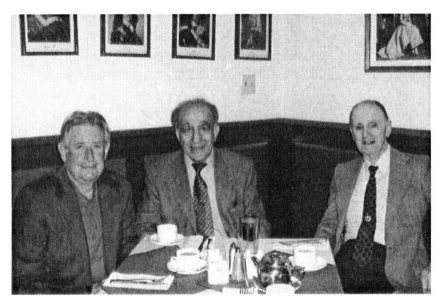

The honorable Ralph Klein (right), the premier of Alberta, Canada, George Abouna, MD, and Rod Sykes, the former Mayor of Calgary, Calgary, Canada, 2004.

Chapter 15

The First Middle East Tour

1977

Despite the desperate situation in Calgary, George built a respectable reputation in the Middle East. The news that the first successful liver transplant in western Canada was performed by an Iraqi surgeon was good enough for many Arab ambassadors in Ottawa between 1976 and 1977 to call George and congratulate him. In fact, he received official invitations to visit several Arab countries. But the most exciting and the most waited for was from the President of Iraq, the late Ahmad Hassan Al-Baker[25]. The invitation was gladly accepted, because he had been away from home for more than a quarter of a century. George was given an official welcome at Baghdad International Airport as the guest of the president. He was a bit surprised to see himself accompanied by a convoy of republican guards and armored vehicles. When he asked what that was all about, he was told that it was for his protection!

A few days later, George met with the president for almost 30 minutes. He remembers Al-Baker as a pleasant man who showed a lot of pride in his achievements. George was given an open invitation to stay in Iraq with literally no restrictions. It is interesting that, after the meeting was over, George was asked by his cousin, Dr. Najeeb Abouna, a pediatrician working for the Iraqi Army, whether he had met Saddam Hussein. George denied and asked who Saddam was. Najeeb replied,"He is the Vice President, but he is the one who is running the show!" As we all know, time has confirmed that notion.

Baghdad looked very different from the time George had left to England—it was now a modernized city with high-rise buildings, modern highways, and an improved infrastructure for public services. He was surprised to see the tremendous expansion and modernization of Iraqi colleges and universities. Medical education and health care delivery were

---

[25] **Ahmad Hassan Al-Baker (1914-1982);**
The 4th President of Iraq since the assassination of the Iraqi Monarch, King Faisal the second in 1958. A leading member of the al-Ba'ath party, he orchestrated the 1963 coup and was in turn deposed by another coup the same year. A third coup brought him back to power in 1968. It is believed that he was forced to resign in 1979 and was succeeded by Saddam Hussein. Many believe that his death in 1982 was the result of a fowel play.

no exception. Every little village and every person in Iraq was covered by the National Health Care Insurance, a totally different picture form the time he was a child when even people living in the capital could not afford health care.

When he was in Baghdad, George was reunited with his family for the first time since he left Iraq. His father was already dead, but his mother and sister were still alive. These moments proved to be so emotional that no words could describe them. George enjoyed every moment he could spend with them and the rest of the Abouna family during his 10-day visit to Iraq. He was able to pay a short visit to his birthplace in Elkosh, where he was reunited and able to reminisce with his childhood friends.

Kuwait was the next stop in his tour. During his visit, he was impressed by the will and support of the government to start pioneer programs in surgey and organ transplantation in Kuwait. George sensed that he would be much appreciated if he accepted the task, a possibility that he never ruled out. A few months later, he found out that moving to Kuwait might be the only salvage for his career, which had been so battered in Calgary.

In 1978 and before moving to Kuwait, George Abouna married Cathy Wade, adding two step-children to his family: Wade, and Carla. Within a year, the new couple was blessed by the birth of their first daughter, Sarah, in 1979, and their first boy, Adam, in 1981.

Chapter 16

Faculty of Medicine, University of Kuwait
Kuwait City, Kuwait
1978–1990

In 1978, the Faculty of Medicine, University of Kuwait, was still in its infancy. The newly established college was looking for world-class faculty members to recruit. One such member was Dr. Abouna. His prior accomplishments in UK, USA, and Canada were highly revered in the Middle East and the Arab world. He accepted an offer to become the founding Professor and Chair of the newly established Department of Surgery.

In Kuwait there was a lot to be done. Modernizing Middle Eastern medicine proved to be a difficult task. Many hurdles were encountered. But the endless support of the Deans of the faculty, Dr. Muhsen Abdulrazzak, and subsequently Dr. Abdullatif A. Al-Bader, and Dr. Abdul Rahman Al-Awadi, the Minister of Health, was invaluable in getting the department off the ground. As chirman of surgery, George recruited many prominent faculty members in different specialties from several countries of the world. George was also instrumental in developing the undergraduate surgery curriculum and the surgery postgraduate training program in Kuwait, an experience that subsequently expanded under his leadership to become the Arab Board of Surgery in 1981, which was adopted by many Arab countries in the region. He served as its first president. This was the time when I met George for the first time as a medical student at the Medical College of Baghdad University.

In the midst of all his administrative and teaching duties, George did not forget his passion, transplantation surgery. He was able to start a small transplant unit of only four beds. In less than a year, he performed his first renal transplant in Kuwait in March 1979, which was soon followed by nine more during the same year, two of which were performed on physicians. But the availability of organs was, and still is, the biggest problem facing transplantation in the Middle East. Most transplanted organs came from family members or form cadaver organs imported from outside, which were of inferior quality, having been rejected in their country of origin. In a society where myths and superstitions are so deeply entrenched in its culture, organ donation after death was almost unheard of. George realized early on that, for his program to be successful, he had to change the way society looked at organ donation. He decided to approach the problem through the religious leadership, taking advantage of a prior experience with the Roman Catholic Church. In 1978, George, along with other members of the International Transplantation Society, met Pope John Paul I at the Vatican, where the Pope declared publicly, for the first time, that the Roman Catholic Church would endorse transplantation[26]. This was later strongly endorsed by Pope John Paul II in 1992 when George met with him in Rome[27]

As a result of persistent efforts by members of the transplant team, several events took place that had an important impact on cadaveric organ donation, not only in Kuwait but also in the rest of the Middle East, if not the entire Islamic world. In 1979, a milestone religious ruling was issued by the Islamic Fatwa Committee of Kuwait that declared, "If the donor is dead, it is permissible to take his organs whether or not he had so willed, providing there is dire necessity..." On the basis of this declaration, the Government of Kuwait enacted a law that made it possible to remove kidneys from cadavers for transplantation in 1983. This was later followed by Saudi Arabia and other Islamic countries in the Middle East. In 1986, a new and more comprehensive legislation was enacted that made it possible to remove all organs from cadavers after diagnosis of brain death, if they had a signed donor card or their relatives gave permission.

Despite the small number of cases performed initially, the Kuwaiti transplant program was considered to be a pioneer in the region. It expended its services by incorporating bone marrow transplantation after George returned from a three-month sabbatical at the Hutchinson Cancer Center, Seattle, where he worked with Dr. Donald Thomas, a Nobel prize–winning bone marrow transplant surgeon. In 1983, George performed the first such operation in Kuwait and the Middle East. It is interesting that, in less than three years after George's arrival in Kuwait, his work was so highly appreciated that Muhammad Msa'ed Al-Saleh, the Kuwaiti Minister of Higher Education questioned—in a newspaper column—whether the government did anything to encourage George and people like him to

---

[26] **John Paul I (Albino Luciani) (1912-1978);**
The first Pope to bear two names, John Paul I died 34 days after his election, making his the shortest pontificate since Leo XI's in the April of 1605.

[27] **John Paul II (1920 -)**
Pope John Paul II, originally Karol Jozef Wojtyla, was born in Krakow, southern Poland. In 1978 at age of 58 he was elected and inaugurated as the Pope. Pope John II was the only Pope whose life was portrayed in a comic book (1983). In 1994, he was named the man of the year by Time magazine.

stay in Kuwait short of a small salary and lodging. Granting him Kuwaiti citizenship, he thought, was the least the government could do.

In due time, the unit had expanded, and the number of patients who received transplants was on the rise, reaching 70 kidney transplants in 1983. While the majority of patients were Kuwaiti citizens, some 40% of them were from other Arab countries, India, and even Canada. Despite all efforts to encourage local donation, the majority of transplanted cadaveric kidneys were imported because they were suboptimal or came from old or pediatric donors and had already been subjected to prolonged ischemia time. George had no choice but to use these suboptimal organs. His experience in Kuwait opened the door for other transplant surgeons to follow in his footsteps. In 1983, George and his colleagues reported for the first time in the literature the transplantation of a diabetic kidney into a nondiabetic patient. Diabetes was considered to be a contraindication for donating kidneys. One day George received a phone call from Belgium. The hospital had the body of a young diabetic man who had had normal kidney function. Because of the diabetes, no other hospitals wanted the kidneys. George accepted them. This case, which was published in the *Lancet* in 1983, sent shock waves through the international transplant community. Of interest, in two such patients, there was a reversal of the diabetic nephropathy. Similarly, it was found that kidneys from hypertensive donors, donors with proteinurea, or prolonged ischemia time could still be used with good results and should not be wasted. Pediatric kidneys from children under 5 years of age were also successsfuly transplanted after they were imported from USA and Europe. George and his colleagues showed that such small kidneys undergoe functional hypertrophy within 6 months resulting in normal kidney function.

In 1985, George went on a one-year sabbatical to the University of Minnesota with Drs. Sutherland and Najarian to gain experience in pancreas transplantation. While he was there, they reported for the first time the ability to preserve the human pancreatic allografts for a prolonged time using cold storage; thus, clinical pancreas transplantation was no longer an emergency operation. George extended his sabbatical to become the director of a new department of organ transplantation at Iowa Methodist Medical Center. He established a successful renal transplant program for central Iowa. However, he had to return to Kuwait to establish a major organ transplant center which he designed consisting of 36 beds with all laboratory and operating room facilities. This major transplant center which was opened in 1988 is one of the largest centers in the world and was endowed by a Kuwaiti family "Al-Essa". It was named the Hamed Al-Essa Organ Transplant Center in memeory of their son Hamed who died after a failed kidney transplant carried out in Europe before Goerge arrived to Kuwait.

Once back in Kuwait, George started a pancreas transplantation program. In 1989, he was successful in performing the first living-donor pancreas transplant in the world outside the United States on a 49-year-old diabetic patient who received part of the pancreas from his brother. He also performed the first combined kidney-pancreas transplantation from a cadaver outside United States and Europe on a 22-year-old diabetic with renal failure. The Hamed AL-Essa Transplant Center was ransacked after the tragic invasion of Kuwait by Saddam Hussein[28] of Iraq.

By 1990, the center had performed successful transplantation of 560 kidneys, 6 bone marrows, 3 pancreases—a record achievement for the region. Of the kidney transplants, 314 were carried out freely for humanistic reasons for patients who came to Kuwait from different Arab countries accompanied by their live-donors. For this humanistic accomplishment George was awarded the Albert Schweitzer Gold medal by the Polish Academy of Medicine in 2000; the first North American Surgeon to receive such an honor. His services were also invaluable in establishing renal transplant programs in other Arab countries including Syria, Iraq, Algeria, Tunisia, Sudan, and Morocco. In addition, he established the Middle East Society for Organ Transplantation, for which he served as president.

While in Kuwait, George was the surgeon to the royal family. He performed important surgical procedures on one sister (Amthal) and three of the wives of the Amir, Sheikh Jaber Al-Sabah; on the Foreign Minister, Sheikh Sabah Al-Ahmad Al-Sabah who is now the Prime Minister. He also carried out kidney transplantation on another member of the royal family and the wife of the Mayor of the city of Kuwait. However, the occupation of Kuwait forced George to relocate and to leave behind unfinished business. His dream of establishing a Middle East Organization for the procurement and sharing of cadaver organs among the different centers in the Middle East never saw the light, and his war against the deplorable practice of trading in human organs had just started. When he left Kuwait, he took nothing with him but his vivid memories, which will always be cherished. In a telephone interview, Dr. Abdullatif Al-Bader, the former Dean of the

---

[28] **Saddam Hussein (1937 -);**
The 5th president of Iraq succeeding Ahmad Hassan Al-Baker in 1979. He needs no introduction for his deeds. He was deposed by the Uinted States and was captured on December 13th, 2003 after several months in the hiding. Currently, he is in US custody awaiting trial in Iraq.

Faculty of Medicine in Kuwait, remembers George as a fine surgeon and humble educator who had left his marks on modern medicine in Kuwait.

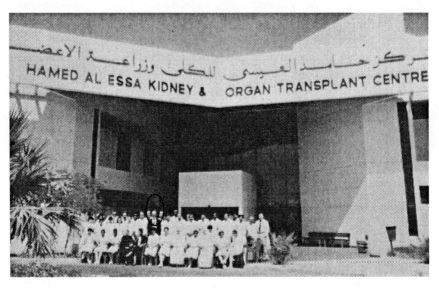

George Abouna with his transplant team at the Hamed Al-Essa Kidney and organ transplant center, Kuwait.

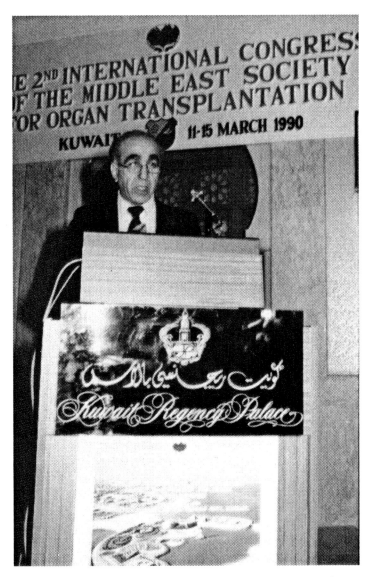

George Abouna at the opening ceremony of the 2nd international congress of the Middle East Society for organ transplantation, Kuwait, 1990.

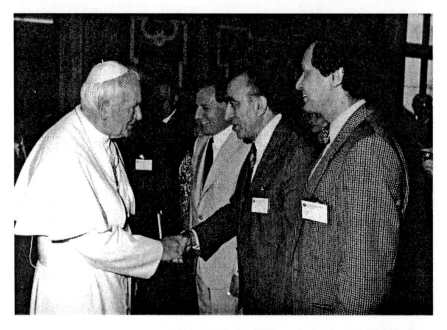

George Abouna and other transplant surgeons meeting with Pope John
Paul II, Rome, 1992.

Chapter 17
Hahnemann University
Philadelphia, USA
1990–1995

While George was in the United States with his family to speak at an international transplant conference, Kuwait was invaded, and the region's largest transplant center was ransacked. The Abouna family lost many of their valuables. His liver perfusion machine and some five thousand teaching slides were lost. Most of the staff he had trained over the years had left the country or gone into hiding. George had no choice but to relocate and start all over again. He accepted an offer to revitalize an old and failing renal transplant program at Hahnemann University. He was appointed as Professor of Surgery and the director of the division of transplantation. The old program was invigorated with new protocols and staff, to be able to expand their case load and started pancreas and other transplants. The plan also included extensive research into new transplantation technologies including islet cell transplantation for diabetes that would put Hahnemann's program as the number one transplant program in the Delaware Valley area by 1994.

Within its first eight months in action, the new team celebrated its 50th kidney transplant, compared with only 10 during the same time period of the preceding year. Before the year was over, more than 70 kidneys had been transplanted, 40% of which involved organs that other transplant centers in the region were reluctant to use. When offered kidneys with unusual anatomical problems, George accepted them and used intricate reconstructive techniques to make them viable. In fact, he developed a new technique that allows kidneys from children less than 5 years old to be successfully transplanted into adults, which would grow to meet an adult's needs.

On May 9th, 1992, Deborah Carrea made history at Hahnemann University when she underwent the first successful kidney-pancreas transplant. George had transplanted both organs into her from a child cadaver. Within 5 months, six such operations had been completed, working toward a goal of 25–30 pancreas transplants per year. In less than 2 years, George successfully performed a groundbreaking surgery to preserve an already transplanted kidney. Denise Wallace-Bond was a 35-year-old woman who had received a kidney transplant from her sister some 9 years earlier. The graft proved to be a perfect match that required only minimal immunosuppressive therapy. However, she was then diagnosed with cervical cancer. The good news was that radiation therapy would probably cure Denise. The bad news was that the radiation would destroy her transplant and she would have to go back on dialysis. Her physicians at Hahenmann offered her a solution—a risky and difficult operation to relocate her graft away from the radiation field. Although it was an unprecedented endeavor, Denise knew right away that she would take the risk.

George consulted with his transplant colleagues from other parts of the country, who assured him that moving a transplant from one part of the body to another had never been done before, but they agreed that it was reasonable and perhaps should be attempted in Denise. During surgery, George and Dr. Antoine Jahshan, a gynecologic oncologist, found that the cancer had spread beyond the pelvis. Therefore, radiation would have to be administered to parts of the abdomen as well as the pelvis, so the kidney could not be placed just anywhere. George had no choice but to relocate the transplant into her native kidney bed. First, he had to remove one of the old contracted kidneys and clear the way for the newcomer. Then the transplant was excised from its current location and replanted into the new bed. The graft was so embedded after 9 years of her initial surgery that removal proved to be very challenging. After 20 hours of surgery, the task was completed with no complications, and the risk paid off. Denise retained her normal functioning graft after 6 weeks of external radiation therapy and a radiation implant. This was published in *Transplantation* in 1994.

While he was still at Hahnemann, George maintained close ties with Middle Eastern transplant institutions. He was an invited speaker at many conferences and had visited several countries in the Middle East to help renovate and upgrade their programs. He had met with and gained the support of the leadership there. In 1994, George met with the Kuwaiti Minister of the Royal Affairs, Sheikh Nasser Al-Sabah, to help reestablish the Kuwaiti transplantation program; with Bahrain's Prime Minister, Sheikh Khalifa Bin Sulman Al-Khlifa; and with the President of Arabian Gulf University, Dr. Abulallah Al-Rifae. This served a platform for a second career in the Middle East. Given the fact that Hahenmann was going through financial crises, George was recruited by the Arabian Gulf University as the Dean of the Faculty of Medicine and the Chairman of the Department of Surgery.

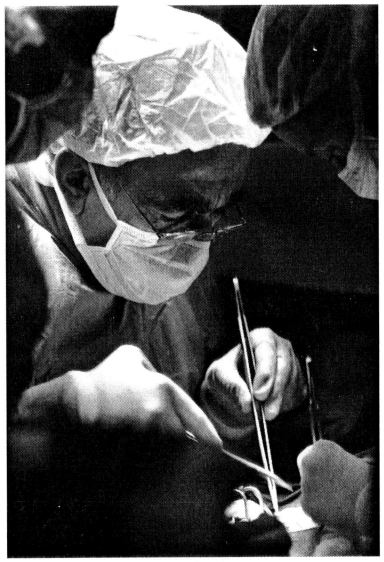

George Abouna operating at Hahnemann University (Courtesy of Drexel University).

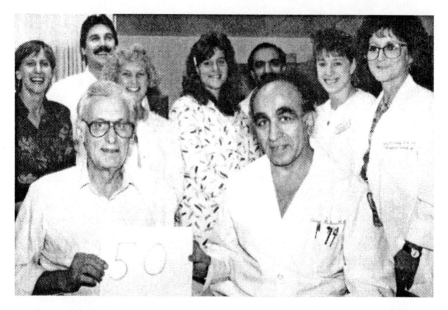

Members of the transplant team headed by George Abouna with Paul Graybill, his 50th renal transplant recipient at Hahnemann University (Courtesy of Drexel University).

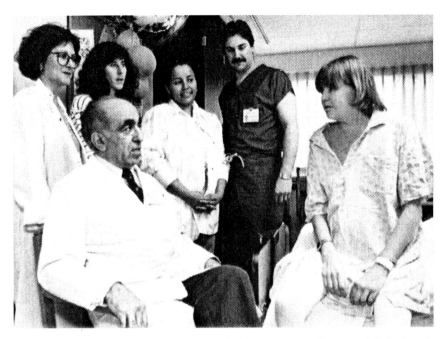

Members of the transplant team headed by George Abouna with Deborah Carrea, Hahenmann's 1st pancreas/kidney recipient (Courtesy of Drexel University).

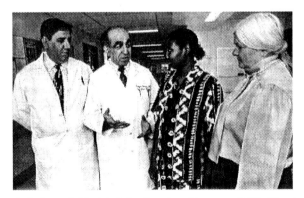

Antoine Jahshan, MD (right), George Abouna, MD, Denise Wallace-Bond (patient), and Patricia Lyons, MD at Hanhmann University (Courtesy of Drexel University).

Chapter 18

College of Medicine and Medical Sciences
Arabian Gulf University
Manama, Bahrain
1995–1999

George went on a two-year of leave of absence from Hahenmann University and accepted his new position as the Dean of the College of Medicine and Medical Sciences, Chairman, and Professor of Surgery at the Arabian Gulf University in Manama[29], Bahrain. As expected, there was a lot for George to do on both the administrative and the clinical fronts. The reforms envisioned for the college required Dr. Abdullah Al-Refai, the president of the university, to ask George to renew his position for another two years.

During his term, George and his newly assembled team introduced many fundamental and much-needed renovations in the college. They created the offices of 6 vice deans and 12 departmental chairs. Entrance examinations and interviews for applicants to the medical school were introduced. The medical curriculum was consolidated to take place over six years instead of seven. The curriculum was revised and updated to focus on a problem-solving approach. Evaluation systems for the students, faculty, and curriculum were introduced. Finally, a performance-based, integrated, direct-observation clinical encounter examination was introduced to replace the traditional long and short case examinations. These changes resulted in improved student performance and satisfaction. The attrition rate in the final examination dropped from 24% in 1995 to less than 4% in 1998.

On the clinical front, George assembled a small team of physicians—a nephrologist and a psychiatrist, in addition to nurses, coordinators, and social workers—and started a small renal transplant team in Sulmaniya Medical Complex in collaboration with the Ministry of Health. As expected, there were many hurdles in the way, the most serious of which

---

[29] **Arabian Gulf University;**
Although established in Manama in 1984, it was not until the fall of 1989 that the first faculty, the College of Medicine, was operational.

was organ availability. Most of the transplanted organs were living donor kidneys. The team had lobbied relentlessly for legislation that would allow the procurement of organs from brain-dead patients. In fact, such legislation was only passed in Bahrain in 1998, setting the stage for more renal transplants.

One of the most interesting cases was a renal transplant on a 2-year-old girl who received a kidney from her father. It was the first such transplant in Bahrain. Mariam Hassan Ali Yousif had congenital nephrotic syndrome and posed a challenge because of her small size. She weighed only 10 kg when she received her transplant. Another rare case was a renal transplant in a 42-year-old man with scleroderma who received a kidney from his brother. At that time, there had been only 20 patients with scleroderma who had received kidney transplants worldwide.

The busy administrative and clinical schedule did not sway George from research. One such project was to rebuild another hepatic perfusion machine as a replacement for the one he lost in Kuwait. With the support of DIDECO Company of Mirandola, Italy, a new refined machine was built and was called the"Abouna/Costa Apparatus." Experimental work in animals confirmed the effectiveness of the apparatus. The device was then transferred into clinical application. Another project was coming up with innovative ways of increasing organ availability. Compiling his own experience with that of transplant surgeons worldwide, George advocated a better use of resources. In a landmark article published in *Transplantation Proceedings* in 1997, he rejected the practice of discarding suboptimal organs. He showed that donor age, diabetes, and the presence of multiple arteries should not be considered contraindications for transplantation. Kidneys from donors without heartbeats and with long ischemia times can be used if the kidneys are preserved by pulsatile perfusion. ABO-incompatible organs can be used if the preformed antibodies are removed and if the spleen is removed at the time of surgery. By following such a strategy, he indicated, the rate of organ transplantation could be increased by 25%–30%, thus decreasing the number of the patients on waiting lists.

In 1999, George turned 66 and had to step down as the Dean of the College of Medicine and Medical Sciences, Professor and Chairman of Surgery, because he had reached the retirement age in Bahrain. He left Bahrain after establishing its first transplant unit. During his four years of service, he successfully transplanted 56 kidneys and laid the foundation for pancreas and liver transplantation, for which he trained local surgeons to be able to carry out the mission when adequate facilities were provided. In a telephone interview with Dr. Abdullah Al-Refai, the former president of the Arabian Gulf University, he affirmed that patients' and students' admiration for George Abouna has rarely been equalled.

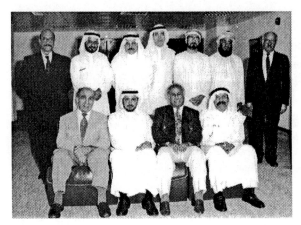

Council of the Deans, Colleges of Medicine, Arabian Gulf Universities during their annual meeting in Kuwait, 1997. Sitting from left: Dr. George Abouna, Bahrain; Dr. Abdulrahman Al-Fraih, SA; Dr.Abdulllatif Al-Bader, Kuwait; Dr. Abdulaziz Al-Ghrain, SA. Standing from left: Dr. Hussain Dashti, Kuwait; Dr. Mohammad AL-Shahri, SA; Dr. Abdulwahab Al-Telmasani, SA; Dr. Talal Bakhash, SA; Dr. Ali Al-Hannai, Uman; Dr. Basdowi Al-Ryami, Uman; and Dr. Abdullah Al-Khars, Kuwait.

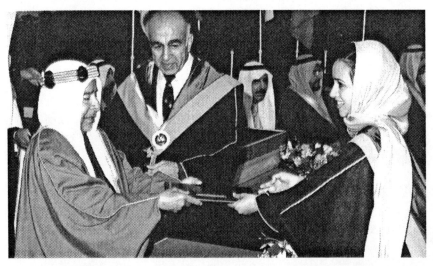

His late highness, Shaikh Isa Bin Slaman Al-Khalifa presenting the certificate to a graduate of the Medical College in presence of the Dean of the College, George Abouna, Manama, Bahrain, 1999.

Chapter 19
Back to the USA
1999–Present

When the retirement age of 65 forced George to step down from his position in Bahrain, he never thought that his age would be a problem back home. Before he left for Bahrain, Hahenmann University was bought out by a private company and was renamed Allegheny University. George kept his academic title as professor of surgery. When he returned, Allegheny was on the verge of bankruptcy. George resigned his position but could not find a job, probably because of his age. He had to take a job as the director of research at Albert Einstein Hospital in Pennsylvania. He was asked to support their liver transplant program with the Abouna chamber when needed and to conduct further research.

A little over a year later, George had to resign his post: the hospital could not afford his salary anymore because of financial troubles. It was around this time when the Allegheny University went bankrupt and was bought out by Tenet. It has since been renamed Drexel University. After the department of surgery was reorganized, George was asked to join them again, albeit on different terms. He was offered the opportunity to start his own private practice within the university; thus, he would have no salary or other benefits except for malpractice insurance. This was a reasonable deal for George, given that he would be able to bring enough patients from the Middle East to support his practice. During final negotiations, Pennsylvania went through unprecedented crises in premiums of malpractice insurance. The average premium of around $30,000 grants increased overnight to around $90,000. This was enough for the university to withdraw its offer of covering his malpractice insurance. George's plans to start a clinical practice fell apart, because he could not afford such astronomical premiums, so had to accept a position of transplant research director with no compensation. It was hoped that the potential use of his chamber to salvage marginal livers would draw enough research grants to support himself and his laboratory. Meanwhile, to make a living, he has been relying on medical consultations rendered to the Physician Review Network and MediMac, work as an expert witness in malpractice cases; and on honorariums that he collects from being invited as a speaker all over the world.

It is interesting that George's initial work during the 1970s has been the basis for reviving some research projects in Europe by which successful trials have been completed to salvage marginal livers that would have been otherwise discarded. Currently, some 20% of all procured livers are considered to be of marginal quality. Such livers come from elderly people, from donors without heartbeats, and those with long ischemia times. The salvage of these marginal livers is based on a normothermic instead of hypothermic perfusion method that is believed to provide a better physiological milieu for the marginal livers to regenerate. If this prediction is proved to be right, it may provide, at least in part, a solution to the problem of organ shortage.

Although George is 70 years old now, he is still as active as he had ever been. He hopes to go back into clinical transplantation sometime, somewhere. His passion for the operating room has not been put off by his inability to afford malpractice premiums, nor has his relentless search for a place in which he can carry on with his mission to the last day he is able to work.

Chapter 20

Contribution to Scientific Literature, Medical Practice, and Education

George Abouna is no stranger to the world body of medical literature. He has contributed–along with his compatriots–a wealth of knowledge in form of 140 peer-reviewed published articles and 33 book chapters touching on various aspects of organ preservation, organ transplantation, and medical education. He has presented 180 papers and abstracts at national and international meetings, and he had been an invited speaker 142 times, visiting many countries all over the world.

George had edited and or authored four books: *Organ Preservation for Transplantation,* Boston MA: Little, Brown & Co, 1974; *Current Status of Clinical Organ Transplantation,* The Hague, Netherlands & Boston MA: Martinus Nijhoff Publishers B V, 1984; *Organ Transplantation 1990,* The Netherlands: Kluwer Academic Publishers, 1991; and *Clerkship Handbook for Senior Medical Students,* Arabian Gulf University: Bahrain, 1996.

He has also served as a guest editor for *Transplantation Proceedings:* 1993, 25(3); 1995, 28(5); and 1997, 29(7). In addition, he has served as a member of the editorial boards of several journals—for example, *International Journal of Artificial Organs, Kuwait Medical Journal, Journal of Medical Principles and Practice* (Kuwait University), *Transplantation International* (Netherlands), and *Transplantation* (Boston, MA), and he has reviewed manuscripts for *Medical Principles and Practice* (Kuwait), *Transplant International* (European Society of Organ Transplantation), and *Journal of Bahrain Medical Association.*

George served on the organizing panel of 12 national and international symposia and congresses addressing organ transplantation and as an advisor to several universities, societies, and many governments in the Middle East. His services for such governments were centered on starting transplant programs and ensuring adequate logistic support for them to be functional and productive. His lobbying efforts were successful in securing government legislation for organ procurement in the Middle East, which was a much-needed step for successful transplantation in the Islamic world.

Throughout his career, George has remained loyal to academic surgery. He was never attracted to any job in private practice. His passion for research and education has been the main impetus for his lifelong commitment to his mission of learning and teaching. He has run many successful departments of transplant surgery and departments of surgery at two universities in the Middle East and led the Faculty of Medicine and Medical Sciences of the Arabian Gulf University in Bahrain for four years. The updates and revisions implemented during his leadership are still alive today, which attests to his wise and long-term vision for the region.

Chapter 21

Inventions

Because of his background in engineering, George has been able to design and invent several devices. His earliest invention was a simple and reusable splint for Mallet finger (*British Medical Journal,* 1965). The splint was made from a spring-steel wire dipped in latex rubber to give it a soft and smooth outer shell. Essentially, it consisted of a straight distal cross-bar and a semicircular loop at the proximal end. In between there were ventral and dorsal semicircular flanges that can be adjusted to accommodate any finger size. When applied, the device will keep the distal interphalangeal joint in a state of hyperextension. Its advantages are its being simple and easy to use, cheap, reusable, having no need for tape or bandage, ability to be adjusted to any finger size, not interfering with the ability to use the hand, and comfortable to wear. The splint was manufactured and supplied by Peacocks Ltd., Friar House, Clavering Palace, Newcastle-upon-Tyne, UK. It was used in a clinical trail of 148 patients, which was published in the British Journal of Surgery in 1960.

This was soon followed by the design of an apparatus for an ex vivo xenogeneic liver perfusion system for the support of patients with hepatic coma (*Lancet,* 1968). Animal liver, through which the patient's blood is circulated, is used as a temporary replacement organ until the native liver is regenerated or the patient undergoes liver transplantation. The Abouna chamber was successful in preclinical animal trials, after which it was introduced into clinical practice. To improve preservation time for the animal livers, the apparatus is designed to reproduce the physiological environment of a normal liver. Within the chamber, the extracorporeal liver rests on a diaphragm that is subjected to intermittent positive pressure, thus simulating normal respiratory movements. An advanced perfusion circuit forms a compact and closed system that connects the patient to the animal liver hosted by the chamber.

The third invention had to do with blood-exchange transfusion. A semiautomated apparatus was designed for exchange blood transfusion for the treatment of patients in hepatic coma (*Surgery, Gynecology & Obstetrics,* 1972).

It has been said that necessity is the mother of all invention, and so was George's fourth invention. George was faced with a difficult situation when he was caring for a patient in hepatic coma. The patient had hepatorenal syndrome. Liver perfusion using his chamber would not be helpful if the renal failure is not addressed at the same time—hence his design for a new apparatus for simultaneous xenogeneic liver hemoperfusion and hemodialysis for patients with hepatorenal syndrome (*Surgery,* 1973). The device proved to be successful in reversing the ailment the first time, although the patient eventually succumbed to her illness.

Finally, George had to replace the chamber he lost during the invasion of Kuwait. The chamber was redesigned to recreate the physiological conditions that prevail for the liver in vivo, including normal hepatic artery and portal vein inflow pressure, total hepatic blood flow, liver temperature, and oxygen consumption. The next-generation chamber, now called the Abouna-Costa chamber, proved to be effective in preclinical animal trials before it was taken into clinical application.

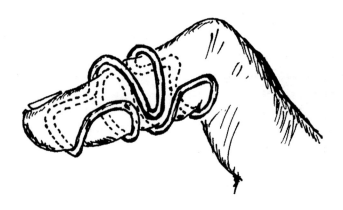

Splint for Mallet finger. (Courtesy of Makram Murad al-Shaikh)

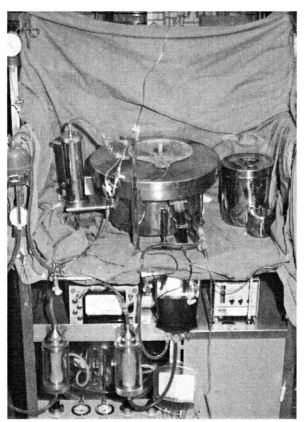

The Abouna Liver Support Apparatus.

Chapter 22

Awards, Honors, and Honorary Memberships in Professional Societies

During his long career in medicine, George has received numerous awards. As a medical student, he received three of the four awards given by the University of Durham to the best projects completed by medical students. He was awarded the Gibb Scholarship and Prize in Pathology (1960), the Dickinson Scholarship and Prize in Surgery (1961), and the Otterson-Wood Prize in Psychological Medicine (1961).

Once in practice, he was awarded many prizes: the David Dixon Research Prize (Newcastle University Hospital Board, 1967); a research fellowship (Newcastle University, 1969–1971); Society of Sigma Xi, Georgia Chapter (1971); and the Distinguished Scholarship of Kuwait University (1982).

George received honors from Allegheny University of Health Sciences for five years of contributions and milestone services to the university (1996); from the Kuwait Ministry of Health on the 20th anniversary of the establishment of the first transplant program in that country (1999); and from the Bahrain Kidney Patients Society for valuable services to the country (1999). He was nominated for the King Faisal International Prize in Organ Transplantation for the year 2000 by Kuwait and Arabian Gulf University.

Many medals have been bestowed on George. He received a Medal of Honor from the Arab Society of Nephrology and Transplantation for valuable contributions to transplantation in the Middle East (2000); Albert Schweitzer Gold Medal for the year 2000, presented by the Polish Academy of Medicine for great merits in medicine and humanism[30]. He addressed the ceremony by delivering a lecture on the humanitarian aspects of organ transplantation published in *Transplantation International* in 2001; a Medal of Honor from the Chaldean Federation of America, Detroit, for

---

[30] **Albert Schweitzer Award;**
Named after the late philosopher, physician, and the Nobel Prize Winner, the Albert Schweitzer Gold Medal is an international award given annually by the Polish Academy of Medicine. The award is also given under the auspices of the Alexander von Humboldt Foundation in New York and is administered by Johns Hopkins University.

outstanding achievements in Medicine and Science (2002); and a Medal of Honor from the Middle East Society of Organ Transplantation at the 8th Congress in Oman, in recognition of exemplary services rendered to the society as one of its founders (2002).

Finally, in addition to his membership in 33 distinguished professional societies, George has been awarded honorary memberships in four professional societies and organizations for his lifelong achievement in transplant surgery: the Sultan Educational Foundation (Kuwait), the United Network for Organ Sharing (Virginia), the Delaware Valley Transplant

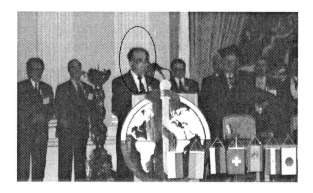

George Abouna receiving the Albert Schweitzer
Gold Medal, Warsaw, Poland

Society, and the Iowa Statewide Organ Procurement Organization.

Chapter 23

Epilogue

Life is a Dash

It may be sad, but it is very true. After the long journey of life, we only get a little dash on our headstones to symbolize our lives and our contributions. Names are inscribed with dates of birth and death, with nothing but a small dash in between. And before we know it, we are already forgotten.

Because we do not know how long we are going to live, we must choose a way of living that will make us happy and proud of our dash. In her book *How to Use What You've Got to Get What You Want*, Marilyn Tam says that by doing so we can ensure our key to success in life. Like many others, George knew from the beginning what he wanted his dash to say for him. Through decades of hard work, dedication, perseverance, and sacrifice, he was not only able to fulfill some of his ideals in life but also to carry on with his mission to the present day: to help those in need, sorrow, and sickness, a mission that often took priority over his own personal and family life.

All I wanted when I started writing this biography was to give George's dash its real attributes. In doing so, I had a few objectives in mind. First, I wanted readers to learn about his childhood, socioeconomic status, education, and the hardships he had overcome on his way to success—in brief, his pathway to greatness. Second, I wanted readers to learn how he reached his point of eminence in transplantation surgery—in this case, his pioneering work in organ preservation and transplantation, as well as the establishment of successful transplant centers in many parts of the world. Third, I sought my own pleasure in discovering the real character behind his personality. Finally, I sought the historical perspective: how has the world changed during his lifetime, and how does he perceive the historical events that have evolved around him, as a participant or as innocent bystander? Of course, many readers may enjoy any piquant gossip about other characters, in which I obviously had no interest whatsoever.

But now that I have closed the last chapter in this biography, I am not sure whether I have adequately covered all of my objectives. The narrated story is only as good as the information compiled. Although George Abouna was my main source, I tried whenever possible to hear the perspectives of those involved directly or indirectly.

I know that, sooner or later, this book will join others under the clouds of dust in obscure libraries*. But until then and as long as George is with us, I hope that we will enjoy reading it for what it is: a snapshot of a surgical innovator and his personal life, while, in the background, we see a past time in British, North American, and international surgery—and further behind—the surrounding world.

* "Medical fame, after all, and at its best, is limited to a very restricted audience. Libraries are crowded with the biographies of soldiers, statesmen, monarchs, orators, scientists, inventors, navigators, explorers, bank burglars, detectives, and philanthropists; and if a library happens to contain a book or two upon physicians, these books will be found tossed unread on the topmost shelf'

(--J. Chalmers Da Costa, 1863–1933)

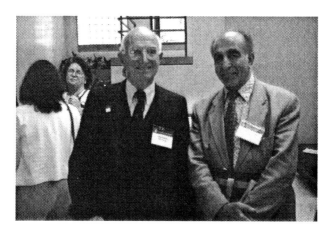

George Abouna (right) with Joseph Murray, a Nobel Prize winner who performed the first successful identical twin kidney transplant in 1954. ASTS congress, 2001

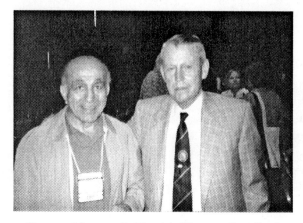

George Abouna (left) with Thomas Starzl who
performed the world's first human liver transplant
in 1963. ASTS Congress, 2001.

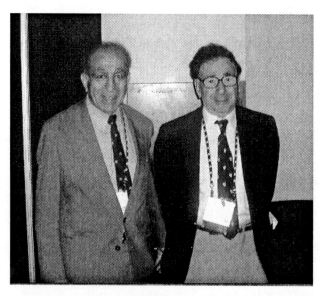

George Abouna (left) and Sir Roy Calne of
Cambridge University-the first to perform successful
liver transplant in UK (1968), The Annual American
Transplant Congress, May, 2004.

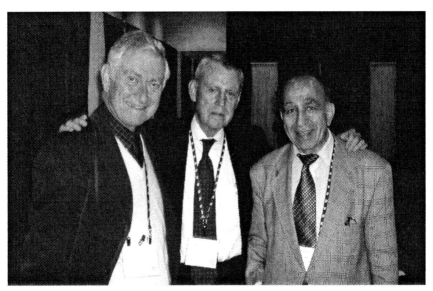

George Abouna (right), Thomas Starzl, and LR Fassati, an Italian pioneer in transplantation, The Annual American Transplant Congress, May 2004.

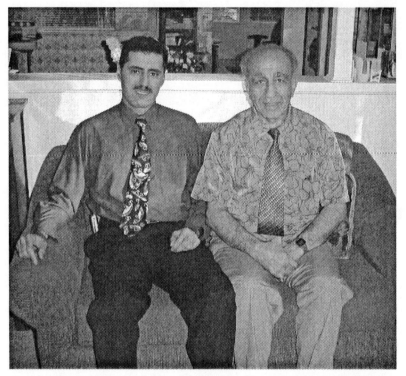

Samir Johna, MD (Author) with George Abouna, MD in San Diego,
California, 2004.

Appendix
CURRICULUM VITAE

Name	**ABOUNA, GORGE J. M., MD, MS, FRCS, FRCS(C), FACS, FRSM, FICS**
Current Appointment	• Clinical Professor of Surgery, Drexel University (formerly MCP Hahnemann University) Philadelphia, PA USA (2000-)
Immediate Past Appointments	• Assoc. Director of Transplant Research, Albert Einstein Healthcare Network Philadelphia, PA USA (Jan-Dec 2000) • Dean, College of Medicine, Professor & Chairman, Department of Surgery Director Organ Transplant Program, Arabian Gulf University, Bahrain (1995 to 1999) • Professor of Surgery, MCP Hahnemann University Hospital, (1990-1998) Director Division of Transplantation (1990-1995) Philadelphia PA 19102, USA

Citizenship	British/Canadian (US permanent resident)
Education **1952-56**	**Undergraduate:** • College of Science & Technology, Sunderland and King's College (Department of Engineering), Newcastle-upon-Tyne (University of Durham)-UK
1956-61	**Medical:** • University of Durham Medical School, Newcastle-upon-Tyne – UK
1967-69	• University of Newcastle-upon-Tyne (Master of Surgery) – UK
Degrees & **Fellowships**	
1956	• B.Sc. Applied Science (Mechanical Engineering), University of Durham, UK
1961 **1966** **1968** **1972** **1976**	• MBBS • FRCS • ECFMG • Georgia State Board of Medicine • MS (surgery)University of Newcastle-upon-Tyne, UK
1979 **1982** **1995** **1996**	• FRCS(C) • FACS • FRSM • FICS

Graduate Medical & Surgical Training

• Rotating Internship (Medicine & Surgery)
62-62   Royal Victoria Infirmary & Newcastle University Hospital, Newcastle-upon-Tyne, UK (Prof A G Lowdon & Sir George Smart)

- Rotating Surgical Residency

    1962-67   Royal Victoria Infirmary & University of Newcastle Hospital, Newcastle-upon-Tyne, UK   (Prof Lowdon, Prof Johnston & Prof Walker)

- Surgical Fellowship (Organ Transplantation & Artificial Organs)

    July 1967 to June 1969 Royal Victoria Infirmary & University of Newcastle, UK

- Surgical Fellowship (Organ Transplantation)

    July 1969 to June 1970 University of Colorado Medical Center, Denver, Colorado, USA

    (Dr Thomas E Starzl)

- Surgical Fellowship (Organ Transplantation)

    July 1970 to June 1971 Medical College of Virginia Medical Center, Richmond, Virginia, USA (the late Dr David Hume & Dr H M Lee)

Certification

- Surgical Boards

    1966   English Board of Surgery & the Royal College of Surgeons of England

    1979   Canadian Board of Surgery & the Royal College of Surgeons of Canada

- Medical Licenses

    1962   General Medical Council of Great Britain (#20224)
    1972   State of Georgia (#014983)
    1974   Province of Alberta, Canada (#6154)
    1985   State of Minnesota (#29714)
    1987   State of Iowa (#26326)
  1991   Commonwealth of Pennsylvania (MD 04351-L)
  1999   State of Illinois (0361010118)

Faculty Appointments

1962-63   Instructor in Anatomy, University of Newcastle-upon-Tyne, UK

(Prof R J Scothorne)

1967-69   Lecturer in Surgery, University of Newcastle-upon-Tyne, UK

(Prof Lowdon & Prof Dennis Walder)

1971-73   Assistant Professor of Surgery, Medical College of Georgia, Augusta, USA

1973-74   Lecturer in Surgery, University of Edinburgh, Scotland, UK

(Sir Michael Woodruff)

1974-77   Associate Professor of Surgery, University of Calgary Medical School, Calgary,   Alberta, Canada

1978-83   Professor & Chairman, Department of Surgery, University of Kuwait, Faculty of Medicine, Kuwait

1983-90   Professor & Chairman, Department of Organ Transplantation, University of Kuwait, Faculty of Medicine, Kuwait

1985-86   Visiting Professor of Surgery, University of Minnesota, Minneapolis, USA

1987-89   Clinical Professor of Surgery, University of Iowa, USA

1990-98   Professor of Surgery, Division of Transplantation, Hahnemann University, Philadelphia, USA (Director of Division 1990-1995)

1995 -99   Dean, College of Medicine & Medical Sciences, Professor & Chairman, Department of Surgery, Arabian Gulf University, Bahrain

2000   Clinical Professor of Surgery, MCP Hahnemann University, Philadelphia, PA USA

Clinical Appointments & Experience

1967-69   Honorary Lecturer & Surgical Fellow in General Surgery, Royal Victoria Infirmary & Newcastle General Hospital, Newcastle-upon-Tyne, UK

1969-70   Surgical Fellow, University of Colorado Medical Center, Denver, USA
            (Dr Israel Penn & Dr T E Starzl)

1970-71   Surgical Fellow, Medical College of Virginia Hospital, Richmond, USA
            (the late Dr David Hume & Dr H M Lee)

1971-73   Attending Consultant Surgeon, Medical College of Georgia, Talmedge Memorial Hospital & Veterans' Administration Hospital, Augusta, USA

1973-74   General, Vascular & Transplant Surgeon, Edinburgh Royal Infirmary, Nuffield Transplantation Surgery Unit & Western General Hospital, Edinburgh, UK

1974-77   Attending Transplant General Surgeon, University of Calgary Health Sciences Centre & Foothills Hospital, Calgary, Alberta, USA

1976-78   Attending Consultant Surgeon, Cardston Memorial Hospital, Alberta, Canada

1978-83   Professor & Chairman of Surgery, Faculty of Medicine, Kuwait University, Kuwait

1983-90   Professor of Surgery & Chairman, Department of Organ Transplantation, Kuwait University, Kuwait, Director of Hamed Al Essa Organ Transplant Center.

1985-86   Visiting Professor of Surgery (sabbatical), University of Minnesota, Minneapolis (Drs Sutherand & Najarian) working on pancreas transplantation.

1987-88   Director of a new Department of Organ Transplantation, Iowa Methodist Medical Center & Clinical Professor of Surgery of Iowa University (Sabbatical)

1988-90   Professor & Chairman, Department of Organ Transplantation & Director of Hamed Al- Essa Organ Transplant Centre, Kuwait University.

1990-95   Professor of Surgery & Director, Division of Transplantation, Hahnemann University, Philadelphia, USA

1995-99   Professor & Chairman, Department of Surgery, Arabian Gulf University & Director of Organ Transplantation, Salmaniya Medical Centre, Manama, Bahrain

Administrative Appointments & Experience

1971-73   Convener of Renal Research Group, Medical College of Georgia, USA

1974-76   Convener of Renal Research Group, University of Calgary Medical School, USA

1974-77   Head, Liver Transplantation Service, University of Calgary Health Sciences Centre & Foothills Hospital, USA.

1978-82   Professor & Chairman, Department of Surgery & Foundation Chairman of the Surgical Department, Kuwait University, Faculty of Medicine, Kuwait

81-81   Chairman, Department of Surgery, Al-Sabah Hospital, Kuwait

1981-83   Chairman, Department of Surgery, Mubarak Teaching Hospital, Kuwait

1979-90   Director of Transplantation Services, Ministry of Health, Kuwait

1983-90   Professor & Chairman of a newly created Academic Department of Organ Transplantation, Kuwait University, Kuwait

1979-83   Chairman, Kuwait Board of Surgery, Kuwait

1983-87   Founder Member of the Arab Board of Surgery & Chairman of Examination Committee, 1985-87.

1987-88   Director, Department of Organ Transplantation, Iowa Methodist Medical Centre, Des Moines, USA while on leave of absence from my position at Kuwait University.

95-95   Director, Division of Organ Transplantation, Hahnemann University Hospital, Philadelphia, USA

95-96   1995-Feb 99   Dean, College of Medicine & Medical Sciences, Arabian Gulf University, Bahrain.

1995-99   Chairman of Surgery at the College of Medicine & Medical Sciences, Arabian Gulf University and the Salmaniya Medical Complex, Bahrain.
Committee Memberships

1972-73   Students' Admission Committee, Medical College of Georgia, USA
1972-73   Vivarium Committee, Medical College of Georgia, USA
1973-74   Transplantation/Nephrology Committee, University of Edinburgh, Scotland, UK
1974-76   Admission & Assessment Committee, University of Calgary, USA
1979-83   Surgical Specialty Committee (Chairman), Ministry of Health, Kuwait
1980-85   Scientific & Research Committee, Kuwait University, Kuwait
1981-84   Committee for the Protection of Human Subjects in Research, Kuwait University (Chairman from 1981-82)
1981-89   Faculty Promotion Committee, Kuwait University, Kuwait (Chairman from 1983-84)
1983-87   Council of the Arab Board of Surgery & Chairman, Examinations Committee
1987-88   Transplant/Nephrology Committee, Iowa Methodist Medical Centre, Des Moines, USA

1989-90   Academic Council, Kuwait Postgraduate Medical Board, Kuwait

1980-90   Transplant/Nephrology Committee, Kuwait University Medical Centre

1979-90   Dean's Advisory Committee, Faculty Council, Curriculum & Assessment   Committee, Kuwait University, Kuwait

1990-95   Transplant   Committee   (Chairman),   Hahnemann University Hospital, USA

1991-95   Foreign Relations Committee of UNOS, USA (United Network for Organ Sharing)

1993-95   Committee for Research on Human Subjects, Hahnemann University, USA

1995-Feb 99   College Council (Chairman), Dean's Advisory Committee (Chairman), College of Medicine & Medical Sciences, Arabian Gulf University and Member of the University Council, Arabian Gulf University, Bahrain Member (ex-officio) of numerous Faculty Committees of the College of Medicine & Medical Sciences, Arabian Gulf University and Member of various Hospital Committees at the Salmaniya Medical Complex, Manama, Bahrain.

Professional Society Membership

- American Association for the Advancement of Science
- American College of Surgeons
- American Hepato-Pancreato-Biliary Association
- American Medical Association
- American Society of Transplant Surgeons
- Association for Medical Education in Europe
- British Medical Association
- British Society for the Study of the Liver
- British Society of Immunology
- British Surgical Research Society
- British Transplantation Society
- Canadian Association of General Surgeons
- Canadian Transplantation Society
- College of Physicians & Surgeons of Alberta
- European Dialysis & Transplant Association
- European Society of Clinical Investigation
- European Society of Experimental Surgery
- European Society for Organ Transplantation
- European Society for the Study of the Liver

- International Pancreas & Islet Cell Transplant Society
- International Society for Liver Transplantation
- International Society for Organ Sharing
- International Society of Angiology
- International Society of Artificial Organs
- International Society of Heart Transplantation
- Kuwait Medical Association (1980-90)
- Middle East Society for Organ Transplantation (President 1990-92)
- Pennsylvania Medical Society
- Philadelphia Medical Society
- Royal College of Surgeons of Canada
- Royal College of Surgeons of England
- Royal Society of Medicine
- The Transplantation Society

Awards, Honors & Membership in Honorary Societies

1960   The Gibb Scholarship & Prize in Pathology.

1961   The Dickinson Scholarship & Prize in Surgery.

1961   The Otterson-Wood Prize in Psychological Medicine.

1967   The David Dixson Research Prize (Newcastle University Hospital Board)

1969-71   Research Fellowship by Newcastle University (To work at Univ. of Colorado Liver Transplant Program with Dr. Tom Starzl)

1971   Society of Sigma Xi (Georgia Chapter)

1982   Distinguished Scholarship of Kuwait University (Fred Hutchinson Bone Marrow Transplant Centre, Seattle)

1986-90   Member, Sultan Educational foundation (Kuwait)

1988-89   Member of Council (Iowa State-Wide Organ Procurement Organization)

1987-95   Member, United Network for Organ Sharing (Richmond, Virginia)

1990-95   Member of Council, Delaware Valley Transplant Society (Sec/Treasurer 1993-95)

1996   Honored by Allegheny University of Health Sciences for five years of contributions and milestone services to the University

1999-Mar   Honored by the Ministry of Health, Kuwait, on the 20th Anniversary of establishing the first Transplant Program in that country

1999-Oct   Honored by the Bahrain Kidney Patients Society for Valuable Services to the Country

2000-Feb   Medal of Honor by the Arab Society of Nephrology and Transplantation for Valuable Contribution to Transplantation in the Middle East

2000-Mar   Nomination for the King Faisal International Prize in Organ Transplantation for the year 2000, by Kuwait University, Kuwait and Arabian Gulf University, Bahrain

2000-May   Albert Schweitzer Gold Medal for the year 2000, presented by the Polish Academy of Medicine, Warsaw, for Great Merits in Medicine and Humanism

2002-Oct   Medal of Honor, by Chaldean Federation of America, Detroit, MI for Outstanding Achievements in Medicine and Science

2002-Oct   Medal of Honor, Middle East Society of Organ Transplantation, at the 8th Congress in Muscat, Oman, in recognition of exemplary services rendered to the Society as one the Founders in 1987

Extramural Experience

- Examinerships
  1982-90   Faculty of Medicine, Kuwait University, Kuwait
  1982University of King Saud, Riyadh, Saudi Arabia
  1982-85   Royal College of Surgeons of Ireland Surgical Board, UK
  1983-88   Arab Board of Surgery for different Arab Countries
  1984-86   Jordanian Board of Surgery, Jordan
  1986-88   Royal College of Physicians & Surgeons of Glasgow Surgical Boards (FRCS), UK
  1989-90   Chairman, Board of Examiners, College of Medicine, Arabian Gulf University, Bahrain
            1992-98   Kuwait University
  1995-98   Chairman, Board of Examiners, College of Medicine, Arabian Gulf University, Bahrain
- Grant Assessor
  1974-77   Medical Research Council of Great Britain
  1983-90   Research Council of Kuwait
  1984-90   Medical Research Council, Kuwait Ministry of Health, Kuwait
  1993-95   Committee for Research on Human Subjects, Hahnemann University, Philadelphia
- National & International Societies

1985-87	Member of Council, Middle East Society for Dialysis & Nephrology
1986-95	Member of Council, Middle East Society for Organ Transplantation
1990-92	President, Middle East Society for Organ Transplantation
	Advisor to Universities, Hospitals & Governments

- Consultant on Surgical Education & Establishing National Renal Transplant Programmes at:

1982-84	University of King Saud, Saudi Arabia
1983	University of Sfax, Tunisia
1984	University of Tunis, Tunisia
1982-84	American University of Beirut & St Joseph's University Hospital, Lebanon
1985	Ministry of Health, Algeria
1986-88	Ministry of Health, Bahrain
1986	University of Baghdad Medical School, Iraq
1986–87	Tishreen Military Hospital & University of Damascus Medical Centre,Syria
2000	Ministry of Health, Khartoum, Sudan

Member of Editorial Boards

1976-84	International Journal of Artificial Organs
1982-	Kuwait Medical Journal
1986-90	Journal of Medical Principles & Practice, Kuwait University
	Member of Editorial Board & Section Editor for Clinical Sciences,
	(Member of International Editorial Board 1991-95)
1986-	Reviewer of manuscripts for:
	Medical Principles & Practice (Kuwait),
	Transplant International (European Soc.Org. Transp.)
	Journal of Bahrain Medical Association
1990-	Guest Editor, Transplantation Proceedings
1994-	Transplantation International, The Netherlands, Mastricht
1997-	Transplantation, Boston, MA, USA

Inventions

◊ *A simplified and re-usable splint for the treatment of mallet finger.* British Medical Journal 1965.

◊ An apparatus for ex vivo xenogeneic liver support for treatment of patients with hepatic failure. The Lancet, 1968.

◊ *A semi-automated apparatus for exchange blood transfusion for treatment of patients hepatic coma.* Surgery, Gynecology & Obstetrics, 1972.

◊ *A new apparatus for simultaneous xenogeneic liver hemoperfusion and hemodialysis for treatment of patients with hepato-renal failure and for patient support before and after liver transplantation.* Surgery, 1973.

◊ Redesigned the "Abouna" extracorporeal liver support machine, which is manufactured by an Italian company Dideco and recently used in a successful pre-clinical trial in dogs.

Research
* Significant past Research

1967-69 Liver preservation and development of artificial liver support for patients in liver failure at the University of Newcastle, UK. (Supported by grants from the University of Newcastle and the Newcastle Regional Hospital Board)

1969-70 Liver and kidney preservation for transplantation by hypothermic perfusion and further development of artificial liver for clinical use for patients in liver failure before and after liver transplantation at the University of Colorado Medical Centre with Dr Thomas E Starzl. (Supported by NIH Grants and Veterans' Administration Hospital Grants)

71-71 Renal preservation for three days by hypothermic perfusion. Further development of liver support therapy for patients in liver failure using temporary support with primate liver at the Medical College of Virginia with Dr David M Hume. (Supported by NIH Grants and the Clinical Research Centre Programme Grants)

1971-73 Development of an apparatus for combined kidney and liver replacement therapy for patients in hepato-renal failure, and induction of immunologic enhancement for renal allograft by recipient pre-treatment with specific antibody fragments.

(Supported by Grants from the Medical College of Georgia [$30,000] and also from the Hartford Foundation, New York [$122,000])

1974-77   Further work on immunologic unresponsiveness by pre-treatment of recipients with donor blood; development of artificial liver using columns of resin and activated charcoal; and experimental pancreas transplantation at the University of Calgary Medical School.
(Supported by grants from the University [$10,000], the Kidney foundation of Canada [$15,000], Gambro Corporation [$20,000] and the Medical Research Council of Canada [$150,000])

- RECENT RESEARCH

1979-90   Kuwait University
The following research projects were carried out in the Department of Organ Transplantation of Kuwait University by myself or other members of my staff as principal investigators in collaboration with several University departments, both clinical and basic science in immunosuppression, xeno-transplantation, organ preservation and islet cell transplantation and were supported by substantial grants (about $1 million) from the following sources:
i)   Kuwait University Research Council
ii)   Kuwait Institute for the Advancement of Science
iii)   Kuwait Ministry of Health
iv)   Sandoz Corporation   Schering Corporation
        Biotest Corporation   La   Roche   Research
Foundation
        Fresenius Corporation   Burroughs-Welcome   Research
Foundation

1985-86   University of Minnisota
Evaluation of function of human pancreatic allograft after preservation and cold storage from 6-26 hours. Experimental preservation of pancreas autographs from 48-72 hours. Portal venous drainage *vs* systemic drainage in human segmental pancreas grafts. In collaboration with Dr David E Sutherland at the University of Minnesota Medical Centre (Supported by NIH Grants of Dr Sutherland)

1990-95   Hahnemann University

Research in immunosuppression, islet cell transplantation and xeno-transplantation. Supported by a special University Grant ($250,000), UpJohn Co. ($80,000), Sandoz Co. ($30,000) and Sharing Foundation ($50,000).

1995-98   Arabian Gulf University

Re-design and development of the xenogeneic ex-vivo liver perfusion apparatus in collaboration with DIDECO Artificial Organs Company, Mirandola, Italy. A successful pre-clinical trial using the apparatus in dogs with liver failure has just been completed (April 1998) and the apparatus is now ready for use in patients with hepatic failure and in patients awaiting liver transplantation. With support from the University and private donations approximately BD30,000 or US$80,000.

2000   Albert Einstein Medical Center

Project of Extracorporeal Liver Perfusion Support previously designed and used successfully in pre-clinical trials is re-activated for a clinical trial for the treatment of patients in hepatic coma as a bridge to liver regeneration or liver transplantation.

The following research projects were/are carried out:
(a) Clinical Projects

1981   Antilymphocyte globulin for steroid resistant allograft rejection.

1983   Renal bench surgery and auto transplantation for vascular and calculous lesions of the kidney.

1983-85   Effect of HLA Typing, Lewis Antigens and MLR on renal allografts in theArab population. Evaluation of modified Surgiura operation for portal   hypertension and bleeding varices.

1984   Donor specific transfusion (DST) in one haplotype mismatched living donor transplantation - a controlled trial.

1984-85   Plasmaphoresis for treatment of steroid and ALG-resistant rejection and in ABO   incompatible renal transplantation.

1985   Cyclosporin *vs* Azathioprine in ischemic cadaver grafts.

1986-88   The reversibility of human diabetic nephropathy in renal allografts.

1987   Transcervical *vs* trans-sternal thymectomy for myasthenia gravis.

1987   Tissue ATP level for prediction of functional survival of preserved cadaveric grafts.

1987-88   Evaluation of unilateral nephrectomy simultaneously with renal transplantation for dialysis resistant hypertension.

1988   Cimetidine in management of post-parathyroidectomy hypocalcemia.

1988   Development of bio-assay for Cyclosporin monitoring.

1989   Effect of Cyclosporine withdrawal at one and two years after renal transplantation.

1989   Evaluation of the Captopril Test in recognition and treatment of post-transplant hypertension.

1990-95   Titration of dose of ATGAM according to level of CD3+ T-cells in patients receiving renal transplantation.

(b) Experimental Projects

1986   Pancreas preservation and transplantation in the rat, dog and pig.

1986   Correlation of blood and tissue level of Cyclosporin with histological findings in renal allografts.

1986   Islet cell transplantation in rats and dogs.

1987-95   Isolation of pancreatic islets of Langerhans for transplantation in rats and pigs.

1989-95   Xeno-transplantation of kidneys: pig to sheep and pig to goat.

1996-present   Xenogeneic ex-vivo liver perfusion for treatment of dogs and pigs with surgically induced hepatic failure (Director of Multicentre Trial), involving Universities of Pisa, Milano and Modena in Italy and the Arabian Gulf University in Bahrain and using the Abouna/ Costa liver support machine recently produced by Dideco Co in Italy.

Current areas of Research interest

• Immunosuppression and induction of immunologic unresponsiveness.
• Renal, hepatic and pancreatic preservation for transplantation.
• Pancreatic islet cell isolation and transplantation.
• Xenogeneic transplantation of solid organs and of islet cells in large mammals.
• Ex-vivo liver xenogeneic perfusion as a "bridge" to liver transplantation.

Organization of National & International Symposia & Congress's

1981   International Symposium on the Surgery of the Alimentary System, Kuwait
        (Chairman of Organizing Committee)

1982   First International Middle East Symposium on Organ Transplantation, Kuwait
        (Chairman of Organizing Committee)

1983   First International Congress on Organ Preservation and Procurement, Maastricht
        (Member of Advisory Committee)

1985   Middle East Dialysis and Transplant Symposium, Istanbul
(Member of Advisory Committee)

1988   First International Congress of the Middle East Society for Organ Transplantation, Ankara (Member of Organizing Committee)

1990   Second International Congress of the Middle East Society for Organ Transplantation, Kuwait (Chairman of Organizing Committee)

1992   Third International Congress of the Middle East Society for Organ Transplantation, Tunisia (President & Editor for the proceedings of the Congress)

1996   Sixth International Congress of Middle East Society for Organ Transplantation, Limassol, Cyprus (Member of Advisory Committee and Editor for the proceedings of the Congress)

2000   Sixth Congress Arab Society Nephrology and Renal Transplant, Marrakech, Morocco

2000   Seventh International Congress of the Middle East Society for Organ Transplantation, Beirut-Lebanon (Co-chair: Pancreas-Ovary Transplant)

2000   XVIII International Congress of the Transplantation Society, Rome, Italy

2000   XXII Panhellenic Surgical Congress, Athens, Greece

Major Clinical areas of interest and expertise

- Medical education
- Organ preservation and transplantation (kidney, liver and pancreas)
- Transplantation immunology and immunosuppression
- Endocrine, hepato-biliary surgery and portal hypertension
- Fluid and electrolyte therapy and hyperalimentation
- Artificial organ support technique for hepatic and renal failure
- Transplantation ethics

Sabbatical Leave

June-September 1982
Visiting clinical Scholar at the Bone Marrow Transplantation Programme at the Fred Hutchinson Cancer Research Centre, Seattle, Washington. Worked with Dr. Donnel Thomas to obtain first-hand training in clinical allogeneic and autologous bone marrow transplantation.

July 1985 - May 1986 & August-October 1986

Visiting Professor of Surgery at the University of Minnesota, Minneapolis. Working on clinical and experimental pancreas transplantation with Dr E R Sutherland.

May-July 1986

Visiting Professor, Department of Surgery at the University of Pittsburgh. Working in clinical liver transplantation with Dr Thomas E. Starzl and the team during which time 50 transplants were carried out.

July-August 1990

Visiting Professor, University of Chicago, Section of Liver Transplantation with Dr Christoph Broelsch. Participated in several procedures of segmental living related donor liver transplantation and other routine surgical procedures of this service.

September 1995-September 1997

Dean, Professor and Chairman of Surgery, Arabian Gulf University, Bahrain.

Visiting Professorship and Invited Speaker at National and International Meetings

Feb 1969   Department of Therapeutics, University of Bern, Switzerland (Prof Priezig)

May 1969   European Society for Clinical Investigation, Scheranigan, Holland
            "Treatment of Hepatic Failure"

June 1969   International College of Surgeons, London
            "Liver Transplantation and Artificial Liver Support"

Apr 1973   University of New York, Downstate Medical Centre, Department of Surgery
(Dr Sam Kounts)

Apr 1973   Washington Hospital Centre, Washington DC, Department of Surgery
(Dr Karl Absolon)

Sept 1974   International Symposium on Artificial Liver Support, London

Apr 1975   University of Lund, Department of Surgery, Sweden (Prof S Bengmark)

June 1975   Canadian Medical Association Annual Convention, Calgary
   "Organ Transplantation Today"

May 1976   Organ Preservation Workshop, Cleveland Ohio

Aug 1976   University of Munich, Department of Surgery, Germany (Prof G Morer)

Aug 1976   International Symposium on Artificial Organs, University of Strathclyde, Glasgow

Feb 1977   International Conference on Fulminant Hepatic Failure, National Institute of Health, Bethesda, Maryland

Apr 1977   European Society of Surgical Research, Warsaw (Co-Chairman of Session)

Apr 1977   University of Baghdad, Faculty of Medicine, Ministry of Higher Education, Iraq

July 1980   University of California, Department of Surgery, Davis, California (Prof W Blaidsell)

Nov 1981   American University of Beirut, Department of Surgery (Dean Khouri)

Dec 1981   International Seminar on Immunology in Medicine, Kuwait

Mar 1982   International Symposium on Urology, Ministry of Public Health, Dubai

June 1982   Military Hospital, Riyadh

June 1982   Seventh Saudi Medical Congress, Dammam

Sept 1982   King Saud University Medical College, Riyadh (Prof Jabar)

Nov 1982   Ministry of Public Health, Bahrain

Nov 1982   Royal College of Surgeons of Ireland, Jervis Street and St Laurence's Hospitals
(External Examiner for Surgical Board) Dublin

Feb 1983   Mediterranean Netilmicin Symposium, Nice

Apr 1983   International Symposium on Organ Procurement, Maastricht

June 1983   International Symposium on Recent Advances in Transplantation, University of Haceteppe, Ankara

June 1983   University of St Joseph and Hotel Dieu, Department of Surgery, Beirut (Prof A Ghossain)

June 1983   Centenary Celebration and Medical Congress, Hospital St George's, Beirut

Jan 1994   Kuwait Medical Association, Kuwait
(Invited Annual Address: "Current Status of Organ Transplantation"

July 1984   Faculty of Medicine, Sfax, Tunisia (Prof H Salami)

Feb 1985   Arab Health Conference, Dubai

Apr 1985   Algerian Society of Nephrology, International Symposium on Organ Transplantation, Algiers

May 1985   Howard University Medical Centre, International Symposium on Renal Failure in the Black Population

July 1985   Faculty of Medicine, University of Tunisia, Tunisia (Prof S Misterie)

Nov 1985   First International Congress of the Middle East Dialysis and Transplant foundation, Istanbul

Aug 1985   University of Oklahoma Medical Centre, Oklahoma City

Feb 1986   Postgraduate Symposium on Liver Disease, Kuwait

Apr 1986   International Symposium on Optimal use of Cyclosporine, Cairo

Aug 1986   University of Minnesota, Department of Surgery (Prof J S Najarian)
    Visiting Professor "The Living Unrelated Donor for Renal Transplantation"

Sept 1986   University of Iowa Medical Centre, Department of Surgery, Iowa City Surgical Grand Rounds (Prof R J Corry)

May 1987   University of Haceteppe and the Turkish Transplantation Society

Apr 1988   International Advanced Course of Nephrology, Tunis

Nov 1988   First International Congress of the Middle East Society for Organ Transplantation, Turkey

Aug 1988   Twelfth International Transplantation Congress of the Transplantation Society, Sydney   (Chairman of Scientific Session on Organ Preservation)

Aug 1989   First International Congress on Ethics, Justice and Commerce in Transplantation, Ottawa (Chairman of Session)

Sept 1989   Fourth International Congress on Organ Procurement and Preservation, Session on Clinical Renal Preservation, Minneapolis

Oct 1989   Second Middle East Medicare Congress, Manama, Bahrain
    (Chairman of Session)

Dec 1989   First Congress of Gulf Urological Association, Dubai (Chairman of Scientific Session)

Mar 1990   Second International Congress of the Middle East Society for Organ Transplantation, Kuwait (Chairman of Congress and Moderator of Scientific Session)

Aug 1990   Thirteenth Congress of the International Transplantation Society, San Francisco (Chairman of Scientific Session)

Dec 1990   First ESOT and EDTA Congress, Munich
            "Ethics, Justice and Commerce in Organ Replacement Therapy"

Oct 1991   Fifth Congress of ESOT, Maastricht (Chairman of Scientific Session)

Feb 1992   International Transplant Course, Denmark (Guest Speaker)

Jun 1992   National Symposium on "The Marginal Donor" by TransLife, Orlando, Florida

Jul 1992   Kuwait University (Visiting Professor)

Dec 1992   Third International Congress of the Middle East Society for Organ Transplantation (MESOT), Tunis (Chairman, International Scientific Advisory Committee and Invited Speaker)

Jun 1993   State University of New York at Buffalo, New York (Visiting Professor)

Jun 1993   Kuwait University, Kuwait (Visiting Professor)

Jul 1993   Second International Congress of the Society for Organ Sharing, Vancouver, British Columbia (Chairman of Scientific Session)

Mar 1994   TRENDS Cardiovascular and Trauma Conference (Invited Speaker)

Apr 1994   Upjohn Symposium on Immunosuppression, Kalamazoo, Michigan "ATG Induction Therapy With T-Cell Monitoring" (Invited Speaker)

June 1994   Arabian Gulf University, Bahrain "Trends in Medical Education for the 21st Century" (Visiting Professor)

June 1994   Kuwait University, Medical School, Kuwait (Visiting Professor & External Examiner)

July 1994   Surgical Grand Rounds, Organ Transplantation - Current Status. Episcopal Hospital Philadelphia, PA, USA (Invited Speaker)

Aug 1994   Nation Panel on cost containment in treatment of renal allograft rejection. University of Washington Medical School, Seattle, Washington, USA (Invited Speaker)

Oct 1994   Fifth Congress of Pan Arab Association of Surgeons, Damascus, Syria
        "Training the Young Arab Surgeon" & "Recent Advances in Organ Transplantation"
        (Keynote Lecturer)

Oct 1994   First Congress of Syrian Society of Surgeons, Damascus, Syria (Invited Speaker)
        "Current Status of Pancreas Transplantation for the Treatment of Diabetes"

Nov 1994   Fourth International Congress of Middle East Society for Organ Transplantation, Isfahan, Iran (Chairman of Scientific Sessions) "Extra Corporeal Xenogeneic Hepatic Support for Patients with Fulminant Hepatic Failure Awaiting Liver Transplantation" (Invited Address)

March 1995 International Congress on Trace Elements, Tumour Markers and Cytokines, Kuwait University, Kuwait (Invited Speaker)

Apr 1995   4th Congress of Pan African and Pan Arab Societies of Nephrology and Transplantation, Tunis, Tunisia (Invited Speaker)

June 1995   Kuwait University, Faculty of Medicine, Kuwait (External Examiner in Surgery)

Sept 1995   4th world Congress of Surgery "The Negative impact of trading in Human Organs" Kiel, Germany (Invited Speaker)

Oct 1995   Lebanese Society for Dialysis and Transplantation "Current Status of Combined Kidney and Pancreas Transplantation for Diabetes Mellitus and Renal Failure" Beirut, Lebanon

Oct 1995   Meeting of the Deans of Medical Schools in the GCC Countries "The Medical Curriculum at AGU" Muscat, Oman

Jan 1996   Development of artificial liver by a number of Universities in Northern Italy, Modena, Ferrara, Triest, Milan and Torino (Invited Visiting Professor and Advisor)

Feb 1996   Italian Artificial Liver Support Consortium of the Universities of Milan, Pisa, Modena and Triest, Italy (Visiting Professor)

Apr 1996   Arab League Conference on Arabisation of Medical Education in the GCC Countries, Kuwait (Guest Speaker)

June 1996   Kuwait University, Faculty of Medicine, Kuwait (External Examiner in Surgery)

July 1996   Consensus Conference on Xenotransplantation, The National Institute of Science, Bethesda, Maryland, USA

July 1996   Universities of Modena and Milano, Italy - Invited Visiting Professor & Advisor on Xenogeneic Liver Support Techniques

Oct 1996   Third Council Meeting of the Deans of Medical Colleges in the GCC Countries, Bahrain (Chairman)

Dec 1996   Invited by the Universities of Milano, Pisa & Triest, Italy (Visiting Professor)

Dec 1996   Fifth Annual Diabetic Conference of the Bahrain Diabetic Association (Keynote Speaker)"Pancreas and Islet Cell Transplant for Treatment of Diabetes", Bahrain

Jan/Feb 1997   University of Pisa, Italy - Invited Visiting Professor & Director of Multicentre Trial on Xenogeneic Liver Support Techniques

Sept 1997   Association for Medical Education in Europe (AMEE) "Teaching & Learning in Medicine, Vienna, Austria. (Presentor)

Sept 1997   Invited by Hoffmann-La Roche Ltd to attend the 8th Congress of the European Society for Organ Transplantation, Budapest, Hungary

Oct 1997   Arab Society of Pediatric Surgery Congress, "Current Status and Future Prospect in Transplantation", Bahrain. (Invited keynote speaker)

Oct 1997   5th Meeting of the Deans of Medical Schools in the GCC Countries, Riyadh, Saudi Arabia

Nov 1997   5th Congress of the Arab Nephrology & Kidney Transplantation Society, Beirut, Lebanon (Invited keynote speaker)

Dec 1997   2nd Bahrain Arab American Conference & the 14th International Medical Conference of NAAMA, Bahrain (Chair of Session and presented two papers)

Feb 1998   Multi Centre Trial on the Abouna/Costa Liver Support Machine, Mirandola, Italy (Invited to participate and Chair the Meeting)

Feb 1998   3rd International Conference on New Trends in Clinical and Experimental Immunosuppression, Geneva, Switzerland.

Feb 1998   New Dimensions in Transplantation Conference, Florence, Italy.

May 1998   Transplant Biology Research Centre and Massachusetts General Hospital, Harvard University, Boston, USA (Invited Speaker)

May 1998   Harvard Macy Institute Program for "Leaders in Medical Student Education", Harvard Medical School, Boston, USA

June 1998   Beth Israel-Deaconess Medical Centre, Division of Transplantation, Boston, USA (Invited Speaker)

June 1998   Kuwait University, Faculty of Medicine, Kuwait (External Examiner in Surgery)

June 1998   Egyptian Association of Angiology & Vascular Surgery, 1st Arab World Meeting, Cairo, Egypt (Invited Guest Speaker)

Aug 1998   Tom Starzl's Transplant Institute, University of Pittsburgh, USA to deliver Transplant Round Lecture. (Visiting Professor)

Sept 1998   University of Minnesota, Minneapolis, USA to deliver Transplant Round Lecture. (Visiting Professor)

Sept 1998   Albert Einstein Medical Centre, Philadelphia, PA, USA to deliver Transplant Round Lecture. (Visiting Professor)

Oct 1998   University of Halifax, Nova Scotia, Canada to deliver Grand Round Lecture. (Invited Visiting Professor)

Oct 1998   University of Southern California, San Diego, USA to deliver Grand Round Lecture. (Invited Visiting Professor)

Oct 1998   INTERLAB'98 2nd International Conference on Biotechnology, Cairo, Egypt. (Invited Guest Speaker)

Nov 1998   National Transplant Institute of the University of California Department of Surgery, Los Angeles, USA to deliver Grand Round Lecture. (Invited Guest Speaker)

Nov 1998   European Society of Artificial Organs, Bologna, Italy. (Invited Speaker)

Nov 1998   1st GCC Medical Association Conference, Bahrain. (Invited Speaker)

Dec 1998   University of Kuwait Medical College, Kuwait. (External Examiner in Surgery).

Jan 1999   Rush Presbyterian Medical Center, Chicago IL USA, Surgery Grand Rounds " Ex-vivo Whole Liver Perfusion for Treatment of Hepatic Failure as a Bridge to Liver Regeneration or Transplantation" (Invited Speaker)

Mar 1999   Invited to give a symposium to commemorate the State of Kuwait 20th Anniversary Celebration of starting the Transplant Programme. "Transplantation in the Middle East - An overview" and "The use of sub-optimal organs for transplantation".

Apr 1999   First Medical Education Congress of GCC countries in Kuwait. "Medical Education for the Next Millennium" (Invited Speaker)

Apr 1999   Northwestern University Medical Center, Transplant Rounds. "Extracorporeal Liver Perfusion System for Hepatic Support in Liver Failure" (Invited Speaker)

Oct 1999   First Yemeni-American Conference in Sana, Yemen, "Medical Education for the Next Millennium" and "Current Status of Organ Transplantation" (Invited Speaker)

Dec 1999   Kuwait University College of Medicine. Advisor on Medical Education and
Research Development and Organization (Visiting Professor)

Jan 2000   New York Medical College, Valhalla, NY, Surgical Grand Rounds on "Current Status of Extra-Corporeal Liver Perfusion for Hepatic Failure Pending Regeneration or Transplantation" (Visiting Professor and Invited Speaker)

Feb 2000   Sixth Congress of the Arab Society of Nephrology and Renal Transplantation, Marrakech, Morocco (Invited Speaker)

Apr 2000   Invited Speaker, University of Calgary Medical Center, Foothills Teaching Hospital, Calgary, Alberta, Canada "Extracorporeal Liver Perfusion Support System for the Successful Treatment of Hepatic Failure as a bridge to Liver Regeneration or Liver Transplantation"

May 2000   Albert Einstein Medical Center, Philadelphia, PA, USA to deliver Grand Rounds in Surgery "Extracorporeal Liver Support for Hepatic Failure Pending Liver Regeneration or Liver Transplantation"

May 2000 Invited Address for the Presentation of the Albert Schweitzer Gold Medal for Medicine year 2000 by the Polish Academy of Medicine, Warsaw, Poland: "Humanitarian Aspects of Organ Transplantation" (Medal Recipient)

June 2000 VII International Congress for the Middle Eastern Society for Organ Transplantation, Beirut-Lebanon "Extracorporeal Liver Perfusion for the Successful Treatment of Hepatic Failure Pending Liver Regeneration or Liver Transplantation" (Invited Speaker) and (Co-Chairman of Session on Pancreas Transplantation)

Sept 2000 XVIII International Congress of the Transplantation Society, Rome, Italy "Extracorporeal Liver Perfusion for the Successful Treatment of Hepatic Failure Pending Liver Regeneration or Liver Transplantation" (Invited Speaker)

Nov 2000 XXII Panhellenic Surgical Congress, Athens, Greece "Extracorporeal Liver Perfusion for the Successful Treatment of Hepatic Failure Pending Liver Regeneration or Liver Transplantation" (Invited Speaker)

Dec 2000 Sudan, Invited Visiting Professor, University of Khartoum, Sudan, Ministry of Health, To carry out Kidney Transplantation Operation on a Sudanese Patient, Al-Kasim Medical Center, Sudan

Feb 2001 Kuwait University, Faculty of Medicine, Visiting Professor, "Current Status of Pancreas and Islet Cell Transplantation for Diabetes Mellitus", Kuwait

Mar 2001 Arabian Gulf University, Visiting Professor, "Humanitarian Aspects of Organ Transplantation", Bahrain

Mar 2001 University of Calgary, Canada, Visiting Professor, Department of Biomedical Engineering, "Bioartificial Organs for Treatment of Human Disease"

Mar 2001 Canadian Society of Transplantation, Annual Congress, "Extracorporeal Liver Perfusion as a Bridge to Liver Transplantation or Liver Regeneration", Lake Louise, Alberta, Canada

April 2001 Surgical Grand Rounds, MCP Hahnemann University, "Ex-Vivo Whole Liver Perfusion as a Bridge to Liver Transplantation or Liver Regeneration", Philadelphia, PA USA

May 2001 University of Calgary and Foothills Hospital Medical Center, Canada. (Visiting Professor) to deliver Ground Rounds on "The Humanitarian Aspects of Transplantation"

May 2001 Grand Rounds, MCP Hahnemann University, "Humanistic, Biomedical and Research Aspects of Organ Transplantation", Philadelphia, PA USA

July 2001 Invited Speaker and Chairman of Scientific Session at the 6th Congress of the International Society of Organ Sharing and Japanese Society of Organ Transplantation, (1) "The Use of Sub-Optimal Donors as a Solution to Organ Shortage" and (2) "Ex-Vivo Whole Liver Perfusion as a Bridge to Liver Transplantation or Liver Regeneration", Nagoya, Japan, July 22-27, 2001

Sept 2001 Invited Speaker 19th Annual Congress of South African Society of Organ Transplantation, 1) "The Use of Sub-Optimal Donors as a Solution to Organ Shortage" and (2) "Ex-Vivo Whole Liver Perfusion as a Bridge to Liver Transplantation or Liver Regeneration" Bloemfountein, S.A., September 16-20, 2001

Sept 2001 Visiting Professor, University of Birmingham, U.K. Developments in Renal Transplantation and Extracorporeal Hepatic Support, September 24-26, 2001

Nov 2001 Invited Speaker at the 25th Congress of the Turkish Society of Transplantation, Ankara, Turkey November 6-9, 2001

Nov 2001 Visiting Professor, University of Oxford, U.K., to Deliver Grand Rounds on Renal Transplantation and Hepatic Support Systems, November 12-14, 2001

Jan 2002 American Society of Transplant Surgeons (ASTS), Winter Symposium, Miami, FL January 25-28, 2002

Feb 2002   Invited Speaker at the Transplant Grand Rounds: The Use of Marginal Donors as a Solution for Organ Shortage St. Joseph Hospital and Medical Center, Detroit Michigan, February 7, 2002

Apr 2002   Invited Speaker for Grand Rounds: Ex-Vivo Whole Liver Perfusion as a Bridge to Liver Transplantation or Liver Regeneration, at Howard University Medical Center, Washington, DC, April 1-2, 2002

May 2002   Invited Speaker at Transplant Faculty Medical Symposium, Atlanta, GA, May 31-June 2, 2002

Aug 2002   Invited Speaker at the University of Buffalo Transplant Grand Rounds, Buffalo, NY, August 20-22

Oct 2002   Invited Speaker at the 8th Congress of the Middle East Society for Organ Transplantation (MESOT). Honored and Awarded as the Founder of the Society, Muscat, Oman, October 21-26, 2002

June 2003   Invited Speaker at the Combined Congress of the Turkisk Transplantation Society and Eurotransplant Society, Ankara, Turkey, June 24-27, 2003

Nov 2003   Invited Speaker at the 7th Congress of International Society for Organ Donation andProcurement, Warsaw, Poland,November 27-December 1, 2003

PUBLICATIONS
(For complete detailed listing refer to full Bibliography)

1:	Published Contributions to Journals	139
2:	Published Contributions to Books	33
3a:	Books Authored or Edited	4
3b:	Journals Edited	3
4:	Papers and Abstracts Presented at National and International Meetings	179

BIBLIOGRAPHY
George M Abouna

1. Published Contributions to Journals

1:01   **Abouna G M**   "Acute Pancreatitis Complicating Pregnancy", University of Durham Medical Gazette 1959; 54:21.

1:02   **Abouna G M** "Science, Medicine and Poetry", University of Durham Medical Gazette 1961; 55:40.

1:03   **Abouna G. M** "The Origin of Cancer: Facts, Hypotheses and Surmise", Newcastle Medical Journal 1962; 28:186.

1:04   **Abouna G M** "Myelomatosis, Presenting with Acute Intestinal Obstruction", Postgrad. Med J. 1962; 58:468.

1:05   **Abouna G M** "Acute Infection of the Hand - Diagnosis and Treatment", University of Newcastle Medical Gazette 1964; 48:4.

1:06   **Abouna G M** "Splint for Mallet Finger - A New Appliance", Br. Med. J. 1965; 1:1444.

1:07   **Abouna G M** "Experimental and Clinical Perfusion and Hemotransplantation of the Liver", Newcastle Med. J. 1966; 29:159.

1:08   **Abouna G M** & Brown H. "The Treatment of Mallet Finger - The Results in a Series of 148 Consecutive Cases", Br. J. Surg. 1968; 55:653.

1:09   **Abouna G M** "Pig Liver Perfusion with Human Blood- The Effect of Preparing and Flushing the Liver with Various Balanced Solutions on its Subsequent Viability and Function", Br. J. Surg. 1968; 55:762.

1:10   **Abouna G M** "Cross Circulation Between Man and Baboon in Hepatic Coma", Lancet 1968; 2:729.

1:11   **Abouna G M** "Extracorporeal Liver Perfusion Using a New Perfusion Chamber", Lancet 1968; 2:1211.

1:12   **Abouna G M**, Skillen A, Hull C J, Hodson A & Kirkley A Jr. "A Comparison of the Effects of Warm Ischemia and Hypothermia on Liver Glycogen, Electrolytes, pH, and Subsequent Function During Perfusion", Br. J. Surg. 1969; 56:382.

1:13   **Abouna G M**, Kirkley A Jr, Hull C J, Ashcroft T & Kerr D N S. "Treatment of Hepatic Coma by Extracorporeal Pig Liver Perfusion", Lancet 1969; 2:64.

1:14   **Abouna G M**, Ashcroft T, Hull C J, Hodson A, Kirkley A Jr & Walder DN "The Assessment of Function of the Isolated Perfused Porcine Liver", Br. J. Surg. 1969; 56:282.

1:15   **Abouna G M**, Ashcroft T & Young JR "Changes in Trans-Hepatic Vascular Resistance During Prolonged Liver Perfusion", Br. J. Surg. 1970; 56:63.

1:16   **Abouna G M**, Serrou B, Bohmig H J, Amemiya H & Martineau G "Long-Term Hepatic Support by Intermittent Multi-Species Liver Perfusions", Lancet 1970; 2:391.

1:17   Pen I, Bunch T, Olenik D & **Abouna G M** "Psychiatric Experience in Renal and Hepatic Transplant Patients", Seminars in Psychiatry 1971; 3:133.

1:18   **Abouna G M**, Hurwitz R & Serrou B "Organ Preservation by Collin's Solution", Lancet 1971; 1:1076.

1:19   **Abouna G M** "Extracorporeal Liver Perfusion for Hepatic Coma", Lancet 1971; 1:1185.

1:20   **Abouna G M,** Aldrete JA & Starzl TE "Changes in Serum Potassium and Blood pH During Clinical and Experimental Liver Transplantation", Surgery 1971; 69:419.

1:21   **Abouna G M**, Koo CG, Howanitz LF, Ancarani E & Porter KA "Orthotopic Liver Transplantation After Preservation for Six Hours by Simple Hypothermia", Transplant Proc. 1971; 3:650.

1:22   Hume D M, Mendez G, **Abouna G M** & Lee H M. "Current Methods for the Support of Patients in Liver Failure", Transplant Proc. 1971; 3:1525.

1:23   Serrou B, **Abouna G M** & Aldrete A J "Hemodynamic and Biochemical Stability After Total Hepatectomy in the Dog", Intern. Surg. 1971; 55:237.

1:24   Bohmig J J, **Abouna G M** & Pardo J. "Coagulation Changes in Acute Hepatic Necrosis", Thromb. Diath. Hermorrh. 1971; 26:341.

1:25   **Abouna G M** "Improved Technique of Exchange Transfusion for Hepatic Coma", Surg. Gynecol. Obstet. 1972; 134:658.

1:26   **Abouna G M**, Amemiya H, Fisher L M A, Still W J, Porter K A, Costa G & Hume D M. "Hepatic and Exchange Blood Transfusions", Transplant Proc. 1971; 3:1589.

1:27   **Abouna G M**, Lim F, Cook J S, Grubb W, Craig S A, Siebel H R & Hume D M "Three-Day Canine Kidney Preservation", Surgery 1972; 71:436.

1:28   **Abouna G M**, Fisher L McA, Still W J & Hume D M "Acute Hepatic Coma Successfully Treated by Extracorporeal Baboon Liver Perfusion", Br. Med J. 1972; 1:23.

1:29   **Abouna G M**, Cook J S, Fisher L McA, Still W J, Costa C & Hume D M "Treatment of Acute Hepatic Coma by Ex-vivo Baboon and Human Liver Perfusions", Surgery 1972; 71(4):537-546.

1:30   Sonneborn D W, **Abouna G M** & Mendez-Picon G. "Synthesis of Transcopalomine II in Totally Hepatosectomized Dogs", Biochem. et Biophys. Act. 1972; 273:282.

1:31   Hume D M, Wolf J, Lee H M & **Abouna G M** "Liver Transplantation in Man", Transpl. Proc. 1972; 4:781.

1:32   **Abouna G M**, Garver F A, Kogure H, DeLong T G & Andres G A. "Survival of Renal Allografts After Treatment with Polyspecific F(ab)$_2$ Fragments", Surgical Forum 1973; 24:318.

1:33   **Abouna G M** "Simultaneous Hemodialysis and Liver Hemoperfusion for Treatment of Hepatic Failure and Hepatorenal Syndrome", Surgery 1973; 73:541.

1:34   **Abouna G M**, Fisher L McA, Porter K A & Andreas G A "Experience in the Treatment of Hepatic Failure by Intermittent Ex-vivo Liver Perfusions", Surg. Gynecol. Obstet.1973; 137:741.

1:35   **Abouna G M** "The Use of Brachial Arteriovenous Shunts for Hemodialysis", Europ. Surg. Res. 1973; 5:390.

1:36   **Abouna G M**, Kogure H, Sobel R H, Lutcher C L, Porter K A & Andres G A "Massive Early Proteinuria Following Renal Homotransplantation", J. Am. Med. Assoc. 1973; 226:631.

1:37   **Abouna G M**, Garver F, DeLong T G & Andres G A "Survival of Canine Renal Allografts After Treatment of Recipient with Polyspecific F(ab)$_2$ Fragment", Surg. Forum 1973; 24:318.

1:38   Jeske B D & **Abouna G M** "Ultrastructure of Canine Renal Autografts Following 24 Hour Hypothermic Preservation", Europ. Surg. Res. 1973; 5:424.

1:39   **Abouna G M**, Veazy R P & Terry D B Jr. "Intravenous Infusion of Hydrochloric Acid for the Treatment of Severe Metabolic Alkalosis", Surgery 1974; 75:144.

1:40   **Abouna G M**, DeLong T G, Pashley D H, Jeske A H, Ginsburgh J A & Linden D R "Kidney Preservation of Hypothermic Perfusion with Albumin Versus Plasma and with Pulsatile Versus Non-Pulsatile Flow", Br. J. Surg. 1974; 61:555.

1:41   **Abouna G M**, Amemiya H, Porter K a & Andres G A "Immunological Studies in Patients Receiving Intermittent Allogeneic and Xenogeneic Liver Perfusions", Transplantation 1974; 18:395.

1:42   Woodruff Sir M F W, Nolan B, Anderton J, **Abouna G M**, Morton J and Jenkins A McL. "Long Survival After Renal Transplantation in Man", Br. J. Surg. 1976; 63:85.

1:43   **Abouna G M**, Preshaw R M, Silva J L U, Hollingsworth J, Hershfield N, Novak W, Shaw D & Vetters J. "Liver Transplantation in a Patient with Cholangiocarcinoma and Ulcerative Colitis", Can. Med. Assoc. J. 1976; 115:615-619.

1:44   **Abouna G M**, Barabas A Z, Pazacerka V, Kinninburgh D, Kovithavongs T, Lao V, Schlout J & Dossetor J B. "The Effect of Treatment with Multiple Blood Transfusions and with Skin Grafts on the Survival of Renal Allografts in Unmatched Mongrel Dogs", Transplant. Proc. 1977; 9:265.

1:45   **Abouna G M**, Barabas A Z, Vetters J M & Litchfield B. "Prolongation of Renal Allograft Survival in the Dog by Passive Administration of Polyspecific Antisera", Transplant. Proc. 1979; 11(1):970.

1:46   **Abouna G M** "Arabian Contribution to Medical Science", Kuwait Med. Assoc. J. 1980; 14:45-57.

1:47   **Abouna G M**, White A G, Youssef H A, Kumar M S A, Wood F, Lubbadah K, Daddah A & Menkarios A. "Kidney Transplantation in Kuwait - The First 35 patients", Kuwait Med. Assoc. J. 1981; 15:77.

1:48   **Abouna G M** "Transplantation Surgery in Kuwait", (Editorial) Kuwait Med. Assoc. J 1981.

1:49   Awaad A H, Omar Y & **Abouna G M** "Cancer of the Pancreas and Periampular Region in Kuwait", Kuwait Med. Assoc. J. 1981; 15:20.

1:50   **Abouna G M**, Kumar M S A, White A G, Daddah S, Samhan M, John P, Kusma G, & Baissony H. "Kidney Transplantation Surgery in Kuwait - The Results in the First 72 Recipients", Arab J. Med. 1982; 1(8):5-11.

1:51   **Abouna G M** "Organ Transplantation", (Editorial) Kuwait Med. Assoc. J. 1982; 16:191.

1:52   **Abouna G M**, Al-Adnani M S, Kremer G D et al. "Reversal of Diabetic Nephropathy in Human Cadaveric Kidneys After Transplantation into Non-Diabetic Recipients", Lancet 1983; Dec 3:1274-1276.

1:53   **Abouna G M**, Kumar M S A, White A G, Daddah S, Omar O F, Samhan M, Kusma G, John P, Soubky A S, Abbas A R & Kremer G. "Experience with Imported Human Cadaveric Kidneys Having Unusual

Problems and Transplanted After 30-60 Hours of Preservation", Transpl. Proc. 1984; 16:61.

1:54   **Abouna G M**, White A G, Kumar M S A, Kusma G, Daddah S, John P & Samhan M. "Renal Transplantation in Kuwait", Dialysis, Transpl. & Burn (Turkey) 1984; 2(1):1-5.

1:55   **Abouna G M**, Kumar M S A, White A G, Daddah S, John P, Samhan M, Omar O F & Kusma G. "Experience with 130 Consecutive Renal Transplants in the Middle East with Special Reference to Histocompatibility Matching, Anti-Rejection Therapy with Anti-Lymphocyte Globulin (ALG) and Prolonged Preservation of Imported Cadaveric Grafts", Transpl. Proc. 1984; 16(4):1114-1117.

1:56   **Abouna G M**, Kumar M S A, White A G, Samhan M, John P, Silva O S G, Mallik M S, Ahmed M & Daddah S. "Living Donor Renal Transplantation in the Middle East - A Review of 145 Consecutive Transplants", Transplantation and Clinical Immunology by Rouaine, J L, Traeger J, et al. (Editorial) Excerpta Medica (Amsterdam) 1985; 69-80.

1:57   Kumar M S A, White A G, Samhan M, Johny K V, Kusma G, Silva O S G & **Abouna G M** "Donor Specific Transfusion in Renal Transplantation. It is Worth it? Transpl. Proc. 1985; 17(1):1069-1071.

1:58   Samhan M, Daddah S, Kumar M S A, Silva S G & **Abouna G M** "Renal Transplantation in Paediatric Recipients in Kuwait", J. Kuwait Med. Assoc.1985; 19:31-38.

1:59   **Abouna G M**, Adnani M S, Kumar M S A & Samhan M. "The Fate of Cadaveric Kidneys with Diabetic Nephropathy After Transplantation in Humans", Lancet 1986; 1:622.

1:60   White A G, Kumar M S A, **Abouna G M,** HLA, MRL, P & Lewis "Antigens in Living Donor Renal Transplantation in a Single Centre in the Middle East", Tissue Antigens 1986; 27:279-284.

1:61   **Abouna G M**, Baissony H, Al-Nakeeb B M, Menkarious A T & Silva S G. "The Place of Sugiura Operation for Portal Hypertension and Bleeding Esophageal Varices", Surgery 1987; 91-98.

1:62   **Abouna G M**, Kumar M S A & White A G. "Optimum Use of Cyclosporine in Organ Transplantation", Proceeding of Symposium on the Use of Cyclosporine in Clinical Transplantation, Excerpta Medica 1987; 81-90.

1:63   Kumar M S A, White A G, Samhan M S & **Abouna G M** "Cyclosporine in the Treatment of Acute Renal Allograft Rejection", Proceedings of International Symposium on Cyclosporine in Clinical Transplantation, Excerpta Medica 1987; 162-166.

1:64   **Abouna G M** & Adnani M S. "Is Diabetic Nephropathy Reversible?", Transpl. Proc.1987; 19(2):82-85.

1:65   **Abouna G M**, Kumar M S A, White S G & Silva O S G. "Transplantation in Kuwait - A Middle Eastern and North African Perspective", Transpl. Proc. 1987; 19(2):21-26.

1:66   **Abouna G M** "Organ Transplantation in the Middle East - Problems and Solutions", In Haberal, MH (ed): Recent Advances in Nephrology and Transplantation.   Haberal Educational Foundation (Turkey) 1988; 233-242

1:67   **Abouna G M**, Kumar M S A, White A G, Samhan M, Daddah S, Silva O S G & John P.   "Renal Transplantation in The Middle East - Experience with 250 Transplants", Dialysis & Transplantation 1987; 16(2):81-84.

1:68   **Abouna G M**, Sutherland D E R, Florak G & Najarian J S. "Function of Human Pancreatic Allografts After Preservation in Cold Storage for 6-26 Hours", Transplantation 1987; 43(5):630-636.

1:69   Kumar M S A, White A G, Samhan M & **Abouna G M** "Non-Related Living Donor for Renal Transplantation", Transpl. Proc. 1987; 19(1):1516-1517.

1:70   White A G, Kumar M S A, Strannegard O & **Abouna G M** "Renal Transplantation in Hepatitis B Surface Antigen Positive Patients", Transpl. Proc. 1987; 19(1):2150-2152.

1:71   **Abouna G M**, Samhan M, Kumar M S A, White A G & Silva O S G. "Limiting Factors in Successful Preservation of Cadaveric Kidneys with Ischaemia Times Exceeding 50 Hours", Transpl. Proc. 1987; 19(1):2051-2055.

1:72   **Abouna G M**, Sutherland D E R, Florack G, Heil J & Najarian J S. "Preservation of Human Pancreatic Allografts in Cold Storage for 6-24 Hours", Transpl. Proc. 1987; 19(1):2307-2309.

1:73   Sutherland D E R, Goetz F C, Moudry K S, **Abouna G M** & Najarian J S. "Use of Recipients' Mesenteric Vessels for Revascularization of Segmental Pancreas Graft", Technical & Metabolic 1987; 19(1):2300-2304.

1:74   **Abouna G M**, Sutherland D E R, Heil J & Najarian J S. "Factors Necessary For Successful 48 Hour Preservation of Pancreas Grafts", Transplantation 1988; 45(2):270-274.

1:75   **Abouna G M**, White A G, Al-Abdullah I H, Kumar M S A, Panjwani D & Philips E M. "The Late Results of Living Related Donor Renal Transplantation - The Effect of HLA, MLR and ABO Antigen Matching", Clinical Transplantation 1988; 2:15-20.

1:76 Kumar M S A, White A G, Alex G, Antos M S, Philips E M & **Abouna G M** "Correlation of Blood Levels and Tissue Levels of Cyclosporine with the Histologic Features of Cyclosporine Toxicity", Transpl. Proc. 1988; 20(2):407-413.

1:77 Samhan M, **Abouna G M,** White A G, Al- Abdullah I H, Kumar M S A, Panjwani D, Philips E M & Silva O S G. "The Use of HLA Living Related Donors for Renal Transplantation is Justified by the High Successful Long-Term Results", Transpl. Proc. 1988; 20(5):800-801.

1:78 **Abouna G M**, Panjwani D, Kumar M S A, White A G, Al Abdullah I H, Silva O S G & Samhan M. "The Living Unrelated Donor - A Viable Alternative For Renal Transplantation", Transpl. Proc. 1988; 20(5):802-804.

1:79 Kumar M S A, Samhan M, Philips E M & **Abouna G M** "Late Function in 48 Cadaver Renal Allografts Preserved for 48-76 Hours", Transpl. Proc. 1988; 20(5):940-941.

1:80 White A G, Raju K T & **Abouna G M** "A Six Year Experience With Recurrent Infection and Immunodeficiency in Children in Kuwait", J. Clin. Lab. Immunol. 1988; 26:97-101.

1:81 **Abouna G M**, Samhan M & Kumar M S A. "Unilateral Native Nephrectomy at Time of Renal Transplantation is Effective in the Treatment of Resistant Hypertension", Transpl. Proc. 1989; 21(1):2028-2030.

1:82 Panjwani D D, Kumar M S A, White A G, Samhan M, Auger L T & **Abouna G M** "Bone Marrow Transplantation For Beta-Thalassemia Major", Med. Princ. Pract. 1989; 1:142-146.

1:83 Kobryn A, Pacsa A, White A G, Kumar M S A & **Abouna G M** "Are Peripheral Blood Lymphocytes the Source of Elevated B-2 Macroglobulin (B-2-M) in Renal Transplant Recipients?", Transpl. Proc. 1989; 21:302-303.

1:84 Kumar M S A, Samhan M, John P & **Abouna G M** "Chronic Cyclosporine Nephrotoxicity in Renal Transplantation: Is it the Effect of Preservation?", Transpl. Proc. 1989; 21(1):1552-1553.

1:85 Panjwani D, Kalawi M, Kumar M S A, Al-Haj J, Araj G & **Abouna G M** "Septicaemia After Renal Transplantation - Epidemiology and Prognosis", Transpl. Proc. 1989; 21:2112-2113.

1:86 Ruka M P, Kumar M S A, White A G & **Abouna G M** "Changes in the Wet Weight of Pancreas During Preservation in Various Solutions", Transpl. Proc. 1989; 21(1):1372-1375.

1:87 Samhan M, Panjwani D, Daddah S, Kumar M S A, Araj G & **Abouna G M** " Tuberculosis: Is it a Contraindication for Renal Transplantation?", Transpl. Proc. 1989; 21(1):2036-2038.

1:88   Panjwani D D, Kumar M S A, White A G, Samhan M, Auger L T & **Abouna G M** "Bone Marrow Transplantation for Beta-Thalassaemia Major", Med Principles & Pract. 1989; 1:142-146.

1:89   Al-Abdullah I H, Kumar M S A & **Abouna G M** "Islets Transplantation In Outbred Rats Using Cyclosporine", Transpl. Proc. 1990; 22(2):873-874.

1:90   Panjwani D D, Sabawi N M, White A G, Kumar MSA, Samhan M, Philips E M & **Abouna G M** "Post-Renal Transplant Erythrocytosis: Existence of Two Distinct Types", Clin. Transpl. 1990; 4:23-25.

1:91   **Abouna G M**, Kumar M S A, Samhan M, Daddah S K & Al Sabawi N W." Commercialization in Human Organs - A Middle East Perspective", Transpl. Proc. 1990; 22:918.

1:92   **Abouna G M**, John P, Samhan M & Kumar M S A. "Transplantation of Single Paediatric Cadaveric Kidneys into Adult Recipients After Prolonged Preservation", Transpl. Proc. 1990; 22:407.

1:93   Al Abdullah I H, Al Ali S Y, Kumar M S A & **Abouna G M** "Electron and Light Microscopy of Pancreatic Islets of Langerhans Isolated by Trowel's T8 Medium", International Journal of Pancreatology 1990; 6:97.

1:94   Al Abdullah I H, Kumar M S A, Al Adnani M S & **Abouna G M** "Prolongation of Allograft Survival in Diabetic Rats Treated With Cyclosporine by Deoxyguanosine Pretreatment of Pancreatic Islets of Langerhans", Transpl. 1991; 51:967-971.

1:95   **Abouna G M**, Kumar M S A, White A G, Samhan M, Kalawi M & Al Sabawi N M. "Cyclosporine Withdrawal in Renal Transplant Recipients Maintained on Triple Therapy", Transpl. Proc. 1991; 23:1009.

1:96   Al Abdullah I H, Kumar M S A, Al Adnani M S & **Abouna G M** "Improvement in Allograft Survival of Islets of Langerhans by Pre-Treatment with Deoxyguanosine", Diab. Res. 1991; 17:181-187.

1: 97   Kumar M S A, Samhan M, Al Sabawi N M, Al Abdullah I H, Silva O S G, White A G & **Abouna G M** "Preservation of Cadaveric Kidneys Longer Than 48 Hours: Comparison Between Eurocollins Solution, UW Solution and Machine Perfusion", Transpl Proc. 1991; 23:2392.

1:98   **Abouna G M**, Kumar M S A, Samhan M & Silva O S G. "Transplantation of Small Paediatric Cadaver Kidneys into Adult Recipients", Transpl. Proc. 1991; 23:2604.

1:99   Shakir R A, Alldin A S N, Al Nageeb N A & **Abouna G M**, "Myasthenia Gravis in Arabs: Prevalence, Clinical Expression,

Acetylcholine Receptor Antibodies, and Thymectomy,1980-89", J of Tropical and Geographical Neurology 1991; 1:49-53.

1:100	**Abouna G M**, Kumar M S A, Silva O S G, Samhan M, Cheriyan G, Al Abdullah I H & White A G. "Reversal of Myocardial Dysfunction Following Renal Transplantation", Transpl. Proc. 1993; 25(1):1034.

1:101	**Abouna G M**, Kumar M S A, Stephan R, Miller J L, Rose L I, Brezin J, Lyons P, & McSorley M. "Combined Kidney and Pancreas Transplantation for Diabetes Mellitus Using Modified Bladder-Drainage Technique and Employing Paediatric Donors", Transpl. Proc. 1993; 25(3):2232.

1:102	**Abouna G M**, Kumar M S A, Samhan M, Brezin J & Chvala R P. "Transplantation of Single Paediatric Cadaveric Kidneys Into Adult Recipients", Transpl. Proc. 1993; 25(3):2170.

1:103	Kumar M S A, Stephan R, Chvala R P, Brezin J & **Abouna G M** "Effect of Donor Age on Graft Function and Graft Survival in Cadaver Renal Transplantation", Transpl. Proc. 1993; 25(3):2183.

1:104	Kumar M S A, Prior J E, Stephan R, Lyons P & **Abouna G M** "Comparative Study of Cadaver Donor Kidneys Preserved in University of Wisconsin Solution For Less Than or Longer Than 30 Hours", Transpl. Proc. 1993; 25(3):2265.

1:105	**Abouna G M**, Kumar M S A, Stephan R, Prior J E, Lyons P & Al Abdullah I H. "Induction Therapy With Anti-Thymocyte Globulin Reduces the Incidence of Allograft Rejection and Improved Graft Survival in Cadaver Renal Transplantation", Transpl. Proc. 1993; 25(3):2241.

1:106	**Abouna G M** "Commercialization in Human Organs", Rev. Esp. Transp. 1993; 2(1):62-64.

1:107	Kumar M S A, Stephan R, Chui J, Chvala R P, Katz S M & **Abouna G M** "Donor Age and Graft Outcome in Cadaver Renal Transplantation", Transpl. Proc. 1993; 25(6):3097.

1:108	**Abouna G M**, Kumar M S A & Samhan M. "Kaposi's Sarcoma in Renal Transplant Recipients", Transpl. Science 1994; 4(1):19.

1:109	**Abouna G M**, Kumar M S A, Miller J L, Rose L I, Brezin J, Chvala R, Lyons P, Katz S M & McSorley M. "Combined Kidney and Pancreas Transplantation From Paediatric Donors Into Adult Diabetic Recipients", Transpl. Proc.1994; 26(2):441.

1:110	Al-Abdullah H, Kumar M S A & **Abouna G M** "Combined Intraductal and Interstitial Distension of Human and Porcine Pancreas With Collagenase Facilitates Degestion of the Pancreas and May Improve Islet Yield", Tansp. Proc. 1994; 26(6):3384.

1:111   **Abouna G M,** Lee D J, Jahshan A E, Micaily B, Kumar M S A & Lyons P. "Salvage of a Kidney Graft in a Patient With Advanced Carcinoma of the Cervix by Re-Implantation of the Graft From the Pelvis to the Upper Abdomen in Preparation for Radiation Therapy", Transpl. 1994; 58(4):520-522.

1:112   Al-Abdullah I H, Kumar M S A, Kelly-Sullivan D, Ilia H C & **Abouna G M** "Autotransplantation of Unpurified Pancreatic Islets of Langerhans Into Different Sites in the Canine Model", Transp. Proc. 1995; 27(5);2645-2646.

1:113   **Abouna G M**, Al-Abdullah I H, Kelly-Sullivan D, Kumar MSA, Loose J, Phillips K, Yost S & Seirka D. "Randomized Clinical Trial of Antithymocyte Globulin Induction in Renal Transplantation Comparing A Fixed Daily Dose with Dose Adjustment According to T-Cell Monitoring", Transpl. 1995; 59:1564-1568.

1:114   Al-Abdullah I H, Kumar M S A, Kelly-Sullivan D & **Abouna G M** "Site for Unpurified Islet Transplantation is An Important Parameter For Determination of the Outcome of Graft Survival and Function", Cel Transp. 1995; 4(3):297-305.

1:115   **Abouna G M**, Kumar MSA, Chvala R, McSorley M & Samhan M. "Transplantation of Single Pediatric Kidneys Into Adult Recipients - a 12-year Experience", Transp. Proc. 1995; 27(5):2564-2566.

1:116   **Abouna G M**, Kumar M S A, Curfman K & Phillipd K. "Kidney Transplantation in Patients Older Than 60 Years of Age - Is It Worth It?", Transp. Proc. 1995; 27(5):2567-2568.

1:117   **Abouna G M**, Kumar M S A, Al-Abdulla I H, Loose J, Kelly-Sullivan D, Phillips K, Host S & Seirka D. "Induction Immunosuppression With Antithymocyte Globulin in Renal Transplantation Using a Variable Dose According to the Absolute Number of CD3+ T-Cells", Transp. Proc. 1995; 27(5):2676-2678.

1:118   Kumar M S A, Cridge P, Molavi A, Stephan R & **Abouna G M** "Infectious Complications in the First 100 Days After Renal Transplantation", Transp. Proc. 1995; 27(5):2705-2706.

1:119   **Abouna G M**, Al-Abdullah I H, Ilia H & Kelly-Sullivan D. "Comparison of the Effect of Plasmapheresis Using Human Albumin or Dextran 40 on the Survival of Pig to Dog Renal Xenografts", Transp. Proc. 1996; 28(1):212-214.

1:120   **Abouna G M** "Ex-vivo Xenogeneic Liver Perfusion for Hepatic Failure", Xeno, 1997; 4(6):102-106.

1:121 Shazali H, Ramachandran K, Hassan K, Tabbara K S & **Abouna G M** "Predictive Value of General School Certificate Scores", Education for Health 1997; 10(2):245-246.

1:122 Al Nasir F A & **Abouna G M** "Students' Perception of their Premedical Programme at the Arabian Gulf University", J Bahrain Medical Society, 1997; 9(2):112-117.

1:123 Kumar M S A, Panigrahi D, Dezii C M, Laskow D A, **Abouna G M**, Brezin J, Chvala R, Katz S M & Phillips K. "Experience With Transplantation of Elderly Donor Kidneys", Transplantation Proceedings, 1997; 29:3281-3282.

1:124 **Abouna G M** "Marginal Donors: A Viable Solution for Organ Shortage", Transplantation Proceedings, 1997;29:3759-2764.

1:125 Kumar M S A, Panigrahi D, Dezii C M, **Abouna G M,** Brezin J, Chvala R, Katz S M, McSorley M & Laskow D A. "Transplantation of Elderly Donor Kidneys Into Young Adults", Transplantation Proceedings 1997; 29:3377-3378.

1:126 Kumar M S A, Panigrahi D P, Dezii C M, Laskow D A, **Abouna G M,** Chvala R, Brezin J, Katz S M & McSorley M. "Long Term Function and Survival of Elderly Donor Kidneys Transplanted Into Young Adults", Transplantation, 1998; 65(2):282-285.

1:127 **Abouna G M,** Editorial "Current Status of Pancreas Transplantation for the Treatment of Diabetes Mellitus". J Kuwait Med Assoc, 1997; 29(4):394-395.

1:128 **Abouna G M** "Kidney Transplantation From Living Donors - Benefits, Possible Risks and Dilemmas", Kuwait Medical Journal, 1998; 30(2):89-92.

1:129 **Abouna G M,** Al Arrayed A S, Farid E, Awad C K, Sharqawi S A-D & Tantawi M. "Mycophenolate Mofetil (MMF) Immunosuppression in High Risk Renal Transplant Recipients", Transplantation Proceedings, 1998; 30:4077-4078

1:130 **Abouna G M,** Ganguly PK, Hamdy HM, Jabur SS, Tweed WA & Costa G. "Extracorporeal Liver Perfusion System for the Support of Patients in Hepatic Failure Pending Liver Regeneration or Liver Transplantation", Transplantation, 1998.

1:131 **Abouna G M** & Hamdy H, "Integrated Direct Observation Clinical Encounter Examination (IDOCEE) - An Objective Assessment of Student Clinical Competence in a Problem Based Learning Curriculum", Medical Teacher, 1999; 21(1):67-72.

1:132 **Abouna G M,** "Medical Education for the Next Millennium-Experience and Developments at the Arabian Gulf University-Bahrain", Kuwait Medical Journal, 1999;31:230-239

1:133   Tweed W A, Abu-Hassan K. Kooheji A J, Yakub M, Tanwani M, **Abouna G M**, "Anesthesia for Living Donor and Recipient Kidney Transplantation", Kuwait Medical Journal 2000, 32 (1): 28-32

1:134   Al-Arrayed A, Al-Tantawi M, Fareed E, Haider F, **Abouna G M** "Renal Transplant in Bahrain", Bahrain Medical Bulletin, Vol 22(2), June 2000.

1:135   **Abouna G M**, "Ex-Vivo Xenogeneic Whole Liver Perfusion as a Bridge to Liver Regeneration or Liver Transplantation", Transplantation Proceedings, 2001, Volume 33, p. 1962-1964

1:136   **Abouna G M**, "The Humanitarian Aspects of Organ Transplantation", Transplantation International, 2001, Volume 14, p.117-123

1:137   **Abouna G M**, "Emergency Adult to Adult Living Donor Liver Transplantation for Fulminant Hepatic Failure – Is It Justifiable?", Transplantation, 2001, Volume 71:10, p. 1498

1:138   **Abouna G M**, "The Use of Ex-Vivo Xenogeneic Whole Liver Perfusion as a Bridge to Liver Regeneration or Liver Transplantation", Graft, March 2001, Vol 4:2 p. 120-125

1:139   **Abouna, G M**, "Ethical Issues in Organ Transplantation", Medical Principles and Practice, 2003 (12), p.54-69, S. Karger Medical and Scientific Publishers.

1:140   **Abouna, G M**, "The Use of Marginal Donor Organs: A Practical Solution for Organ Shortage", Annals of Transplantation, 2004 Volume 9(1), p.62-66 (In Press)

2. Published Contributions to Books

2:01   Pen I, Busch T, Olenik D & **Abouna G M** "Psychiatric Experience in Renal and Hepatic Transplant Patients", In: Psychiatric Aspects of Organ Transplantation by Castelnouvo-Tedeco. P. (Edit) Grune & Stratton, New York 1971; 133-145.

2:02   **Abouna G M** "Viability Essays in Organ Preservation", In: Organ Preservation for Transplantation by Karow A, **Abouna G M** & Humphries A L (Edit) Little Brown & Co, Boston 1974; 108-128.

2:03   **Abouna G M** "Perfusion Technology", In: Organ Preservation for Transplantation by Karow A, **Abouna G M** & Humphries A L (Edit) Little Brown & Co, Boston 1974; 239-258.

2:04   **Abouna G M** "Liver Preservation", In: Organ Preservation for Transplantation by Karow A, Abouna G M & Humphries A L (Edit) Little Brown & Co, Boston 1974; 349-371.

2:05   **Abouna G M**   Gilchrist T, Pettit J T, Boyd N, Todd J K, Courtney J M & Malni R. "Hemoperfusion With Activated Charcoal in Treatment of Experimental Acute Hepatic Failure", In: Artificial Liver Support by Williams R & Murray-Lyons I (Edit) Pitman Medical Publishers 1975; 180-185.

2:06   **Abouna G M** "Extracorporeal Liver Perfusion", In: Hepatic Support in Liver Failure by Kuster G (Edit) Charles C Thomas 1976; 159-193.

2:07   **Abouna G M** "Cross-Circulation", In: Hepatic Support in Liver Failure by Kuster G (Edit) Charles C Thomas 1976; 194-208.

2:08   **Abouna G M,** Barabas A S, Alexander F, Todd J K, Boyd H & Kinniburgh D. "Animal Models for the Study of Acute Hepatic Failure and Evaluation of Artificial Liver Support Techniques", In: Artificial Organs - Proceedings of Strathclyde Bioengineering Seminar by Kennedi R M & Gilchrist T (Edit) MacMillan 1977; 351-362.

2:09   **Abouna G M,** Barabas A S, Boyd N, Todd J K, Alexander F, Kinniburgh D, Gilchrist T & Johnson E. "Resin and Charcoal Hemoperfusion in Treatment of Hepatic Coma", In: Artificial Organs - Proceedings of Strathclyde Bioengineering Seminar by Kennedy R M & Gilchrist T (Edit) MacMillan 1977; 363-371.

2:10   **Abouna G M** "Liver Transplantation", In: Organ Transplantation by Chatterjee S N (Edit) John Wright, PSG Publications, Littleton M A 1982; 269-327.

2:11   **Abouna G M** "Renal Transplantation in the Developing World", In: Tropical Urology and Renal Disease by Husain I (Edit) Churchill & Livingstone 1984; 67-70.

2:12   **Abouna G M**, White A G, Kumar M S A, Daddah S K & Samhan M. "The Development of a Renal Transplantation Programme in Kuwait and the Results in the First 142 grafts", In: Current Status of Clinical Organ Transplantation by Abouna G M (Edit) Martinus Nijhoff, The Hague 1984; 193-207.

2:13   White A G & **Abouna G M** "HLA and B Matching, The Mixed Lymphocyte Reaction and Renal Allograft Survival in a Single Centre", In: Current Status of Clinical Organ Transplantation Abouna G M (Edit) Martinus Nijhoff, The Hague 1984; 7-13.

2:14   Kumar M S A, White A G, John P & **Abouna G M** "Antilymphocyte Globulin Infusion in Rejection - A Prospective Study", In: Current Status of Clinical Organ Transplantation Abouna G M (Edit) Martinus Nijhoff, The Hague 1984; 49-56.

2:15   Kusma G, Hilali N A & **Abouna G M** "Renal Replacement Therapy in Kuwait", In: <u>Current Status of Clinical Organ Transplantation</u> Abouna G M (Edit) Martinus Nijhoff, The Hague 1984; 187-191.

2:16   **Abouna G M**, Kumar M S A, White A G, Daddah S M & Silva O S G. "Prolonged Preservation of Imported Cadaveric Grafts By Ice Cooling With Euro-Collins Solution Versus Hypothermic Pulsation Perfusion", In: <u>Current Status of Clinical Organ Transplantation</u> Abouna G M (Edit) Martinus Nijhoff, The Hague 1984; 123-130.

2:17   Daddah S K, Samhan M Omar O F & **Abouna G M** "Permanent Vascular Access for Hemodialysis: The Kuwait Experience", In: Abouna G M, ed. <u>Current Status of Clinical Organ Transplantation</u> Martinus Nijhoff, The Hague 1984; 147-151.

2:18   John P, Kumar M S A, Samhan M & **Abouna G M** "The Living Donor for Kidney Transplantation: A Review of 100 Consecutive Donors",   In: Abouna G M, ed. <u>Current Status of Clinical Organ Transplantation</u> Martinus Nijhoff, The Hague 1984; 163-171.

2:19   **Abouna G M** "Renal Autotransplantation and Extracorporeal Renal Surgery", In: Abouna G M, ed. <u>Current Status of Clinical Organ Transplantation</u> Martinus Nijhoff The Hague 1984; 285-295.

2:20   **Abouna G M** "Development of Renal Transplantation in Kuwait", In: Salah H, ed. <u>Proceedings of Symposium Prospectives de la Transplantation Renale</u> Algiers: Institute of National D'Ensignement Superior en Sciences Medicals and Society Algerienne de Nephrologie 1985; 135-146.

2:21   **Abouna G M** "Organ Transplantation in the Middle East - Problems and Possible Solutions", In: Haberal M A, ed. <u>Recent Advances in Nephrology & Transplantation</u> Ankara, Turkey, Pelin Group Publishing Co 1990; 233-242.

2:22   **Abouna G M**, Kumar M S A, Kalawi M, Samhan M, White A G, Al Abdullah I H Kobryn A, Al Dadah S, Sabawi N, John P & Philips E M. "Ten-Year Experience with 500 Renal Transplants", In: Abouna G M, Kumar M S A & White A G, eds. <u>Organ Transplantation 1990</u> Dordrecht, The Netherlands: Kluwer Academic Publishers 1991; 167-187.

2:23   Al Abdullah I H, Kumar M S A, Al Adnani M S & **Abouna G M** "Does Pretreatment of Islets of Langerhans with Deoxyguanosine Improve Allograft Survival Without Immunosuppression?", In: Abouna G M, Kumar M S A & White A G, eds. <u>Organ Transplantation 1990</u> Dordrecht, The Netherlands: Kluwer Academic Publishers 1991; 409-414.

2:24   White A G, Panjwani D, Angelo-Khattar M, El-Deen A S, Kumar M S A, Philips E M & **Abouna G M** "Comparison of Cyclosporine Assays Using Radio-immunoassay, Fluorescent Polarisation Immunoassay and High-Performance Liquid Chromatography", In: Abouna G M, Kumar M S A & White A G, eds. Organ Transplantation 1990 Dordrecht, The Netherlands: Kluwer Academic Publishers 1991; 159-162.

2:25   Kalawi M, Al Sabawi N A, Samhan M, Panjwani D, Kumar M S A, Philips E M & **Abouna G M** "Cyclosporine Withdrawal in Renal Transplant Recipients Maintained on Azathioprine, Prednisone, and Cyclosporine", In: Abouna G M, Kumar M S A & White A G, eds. Organ Transplantation 1990 Dordrecht, The Netherlands: Kluwer Academic Publishers 1991; 101-107.

2:26   Abdul Karim M, Kumar M S A, Samhan M, John P, Hassan I M, Abdul Basit S, Philips E M & **Abouna G M** "Urological Complications in 510 Consecutive Renal Transplants", In: Abouna G M, Kumar M S A & White A G, eds. Organ Transplantation 1990 Dordrecht, the Netherlands: Kluwer Academic Publishers 1991; 505-509.

2:27   White A G, Raju K T, Kumar M S A, Philips E M & **Abouna G M** "Rapid Lymphocyte Crossmatching for Renal Transplantation", In: Abouna G M, Kumar M S A & White A G, eds. Organ Transplantation 1990 Dordrecht, The Netherlands: Kluwer Academic Publishers 1991; 39-41.

2:28   Al Dadah S, Kalawi M, Samhan M, John P, Kumar M S A & **Abouna G M** "Current Techniques for Permanent Vascular Access Surgery - Experience With 930 Procedures", In: Abouna G M, Kumar M S A & White A G, eds. Organ Transplantation 1990 Dordrecht, The Netherlands: Kluwer Academic Publishers 1991; 237-245.

2:29   **Abouna G M**, John P, Kumar M S A, White A G, Silva O S G, Shuwaikh E, Samhan M, Philips E M & Al Dadah S. "The Use of Single Paediatric Cadaver Kidneys for Transplantation into Adult Recipients", In: Abouna G M, Kumar M S A & White A G, eds. Organ Transplantation 1990 Dordrecht, The Netherlands: Kluwer Academic Publishers 1991; 211-215.

2:30   Samhan M, John P, Kumar M S A, White A G, Silva O S G, Shuwaikh E, Philips E M, Al Dadah S & **Abouna G M** "Renal Transplantation in Children", In: Abouna G M, Kumar M S A & White A G, eds. Organ Transplantation 1990 Dordrecht, The Netherlands: Kluwer Academic Publishers 1991; 225-231.

2:31   **Abouna G M** "Moral, Ethical and Medical Values Sacrificed by Commercialisation in Human Organs", In: Abouna G M,

131

Kumar M S A & White A G, eds. <u>Organ Transplantation 1990</u> Dordrecht, The Netherlands: Kluwer Academic Publishers 1991; 545-553.

2:32   **Abouna G M**, Sabawi M M, Kumar M S A, Samhan M. "The Negative Impact of Paid Organ Donation", In: Land W, & Dossetor J B, eds. <u>Organ Replacement Therapy: Ethics, Justice, Commerce</u> Berlin/ Heidelberg: Springer-Verlag 1991; 164-172.

2:33   **Abouna G M** "Extracorporeal Xenogeneic Liver Perfusion for the Treatment of Hepatic Failure", In: Cooper D, Kemp E, Reemtsma K, White D & Platt J, eds. <u>Xenotransplantation</u> Springer-Verlag Berlin Heidelberg New York 1997.

3a. Books Authored or Edited

3:01   Karow A, **Abouna G M** & Humphries A L, eds. **Organ Preservation for Transplantation** Boston M A: Little, Brown & Co 1974.

3:02   **Abouna G M** ed. **Current Status of Clinical Organ Transplantation** The Hague, Netherlands & Boston M A: Martinus Nijhoff Publishers B V 1984.

3:03   **Abouna G M**, Kumar M S A & White A G, eds. **Organ Transplantation 1990** the Netherlands: Kluwer Academic Publishers 1991.

3:04   Hamdy H, **Abouna G M** **Clerkship Handbook for Senior Medical Students**, Arabian Gulf University: Bahrain 1996.

3b. Journals Edited

3:05   **Abouna G M**, Bilgin N & El Matri A, (Guest Eds) Transplantation Proceedings 1993; 25(3).

3:06   **Abouna G M,** Fagil E, Ghods A J (Guest Eds) Transplantation Proceedings 1995; 28(5).

3:07   **Abouna G M,** El Matri A, Kyriakides G K (Guest Eds) Transplantation Proceedings 1997; 29(7).

4. Papers & Abstracts Presented at National & International Meetings

4:01   Methods for the assessment of function of the isolated perfused porcine liver. Surgical Research Society. London, England, January 1968.

4:02   Hemodynamic, biochemical and immunologic observations in heterologous extracorporeal hepatic support. Surgical Research Society, Leeds, England, July 1968.

4:03   Pig liver perfusions with human blood: The effect of flushing the liver with various electrolyte solutions. Associations of Surgeons of Great Britain (Moynihan Prize Competition), Royal College of Surgeons of England, April 1968.

4:04   Transhepatic vascular resistance during isolated porcine liver perfusions. Surgical Research Society. Oxford, England, January 1969.

4:05   Changes in pH and electrolytes following ischemia and hypothermia of the liver. Surgical Research Society. Oxford, England, January 1969.

4:06   Personal experience and techniques in the treatment of hepatic failure. Workshop on treatment of Hepatic Coma. European Society for Clinical Investigation. Schvanegan, Holland, May 1969.

4:07   Long-term hepatic support by intermittent liver perfusions. European Society for the Study of the Liver. Berne, Switzerland, September 1971.

4:08   Successful orthotopic liver transplantation after preservation for six hours by simple cooling. Third International Congress of the Transplantation Society. The Hague, Holland, September 1971.

4:09   A method of long-term kidney preservation. Seventh European Experimental Surgery Congress. Amsterdam, Holland, April 1972.

4:10   The use of brachial A-V shunts for hemodialysis and other extracorporeal support procedures. Seventh European Experimental Surgery Congress. Amsterdam, Holland, April 1972.

4:11   Experience in hepatic support therapy by intermittent extracorporeal liver perfusion. Seventh European Experimental Surgery Congress, Amsterdam, Holland, April 1972.

4:12   Immunological studies in patients receiving multi-species, xenogeneic and allogeneic liver perfusions. Fourth International Congress of the Transplantation Society, San Francisco, USA, September 1972.

4:13   Enhancement of canine renal allografts by treatment of donor organ and recipient with polyspecific homologous and heterologous F(ab)$_2$. European Society for Surgical Research, The Hague, The Netherlands 1973.

4:14   Survival of canine renal allograft after treatment with polyspecific F(ab)$_2$ fragments. American College of Surgeons Annual Clinical Congress, Chicago, IL, USA, Oct 1973.

4:15   Kidney preservation by hypothermic perfusion with albumin versus plasma and with pulsatile versus non-pulsatile flow. Eighth European Surgical Congress, Oslo, Norway, May 1973.

4:16   Critical valuation of viability assays in renal preservation. Surgical Research Society, London, England, January 1974.

4:17   Hemoperfusion through activated charcoal for treatment of acute hepatic failure. The Royal College of Physicians and Surgeons of Canada Annual Meeting, Winnipeg, Canada, January 1975.

4:18   Parameters of cell viability for Kidney preservation. Annual Meeting of the Royal College of Physicians and Surgeons of Canada, Winnipeg, Canada, January 1975.

4:19   The effect of pretreatment with multiple blood transfusions and with skin grafts on the survival of renal allografts in mongrel dogs. Sixth International Congress of the Transplantation Society, New York, NY, USA, August 1976.

4:20   Animal models for hepatic failure. Twelfth Congress of the European Society for Surgical Research, Warsaw, Poland, April 1977.

4:21   Active enhancement of renal allografts by pretreatment with polyspecific antigens and passive enhancement with polyspecific immunoantiserum. Twelfth Congress of the European Society for Surgical Research, Warsaw, Poland, April 1977.

4:22   Resin and Charcoal hemoperfusion in treatment of hepatic failure. Twelfth Congress of the European Society of Surgical Research, Warsaw, Poland, April 1977.

4:23   Enhancement of renal allografts by recipient treatment with immune alloantisera. International Congress of the Transplantation Society. Rome, Italy, September 1978.

4:24   **Abouna G M,** White A G, Youssef A H, et al. Kidney transplantation in Kuwait. First International Conference of Kuwait University. Kuwait, January 1981.

4:25   **Abouna G M,** Kumar A S, Lubbadah M K, et al. Acute renal allografts rejection successfully treated with intravenous and antilymphocyte globulin (ALG). First International Conference of Kuwait University, Kuwait, January 1981.

4:26   Awaad A H, Yazgi M, Omar Y, Barakat M & **Abouna G M.** Cancer of pancreas and periampullary region. First International Conference of Kuwait University, Kuwait, January 1981.

4:27   Alwan M H, Menkarios A, Mullick R J, Barat M, Menon K & **Abouna G M.** Hydatid disease of the liver in Kuwait. First International Conference of Kuwait University, Kuwait, January 1981.

4:28   Menkarios A, Alwan A, Kumar M S A, Baissoni H, Barakat M, Badawi A & **Abouna G M.** Distal splenorenal shunt for portal hypertension. First International Conference of Kuwait University, Kuwait, January 1981.

4:29   **Abouna G M.** Operable cancer of the breast. International Symposium on Oncology and Chemotherapy, Kuwait, February 1981.

4:30   **Abouna G M.** Immunosuppression. International Seminar on Immunology in Medicine, Kuwait, December 1981.

4:31   **Abouna G M.** Intravenous ALG in treatment of acute renal allografts rejection. American Society of Transplant Surgeons, Chicago, IL, USA, June 1981.

4:32   **Abouna G M**, Menkarios A, Youssef A H, Al Naqueeb B & Farooq O. Early experience in the surgical treatment of portal hypertension in Kuwait. International Symposium on Surgery of the Alimentary System, Kuwait, February 1982.

4:33   Alwan M, **Abouna G M.** Hydatid disease in Kuwait. International Symposium on Surgery of the Alimentary System, Kuwait, February 1982.

4:34   **Abouna G M.** Extracorporeal renal surgery. International Urology Symposium, Department of Health and Medical Services, Dubai, UAE, March 1982.

4:35   **Abouna G M.** Kidney transplantation - current status. International Urology Symposium, Department of Health and Medical Services, Dubai, UAE, March 1982.

4:36   **Abouna G M.** Experience with 72 renal transplants in Kuwait. Seventh Saudi Medical Congress, Dammam, Saudi Arabia, June 1982.

4:37   **Abouna G M,** Samhan M, Kumar M S A, John P, Daddah S & Kusma G. Renal transplantation in paediatric patients. Sixth Mediterranean Paediatric Congress, Kuwait, September 1982.

4:38   **Abouna G M,** Omar O F, Kumar M S A, Haj K E & Bahri A. Netilmicin in kidney transplant and immunosuppressed patients. Mediterranean Symposium on Aminoglycoside, Nice, France 1983.

4:39   **Abouna G M,** Kumar M S A, White A G, Daddah S, Omar O F, Samhan M, Kusma G, John P, Soubky A S, Abbas A R & Kremer G. Experience with imported human cadaveric kidneys having unusual problems and transplanted after 30-60 hours of preservation. International Congress on Organ Procurement, Maastricht, Holland, April 1983.

4:40   **Abouna G M,** Kumar M S A, White A G, et al. Experience with 130 consecutive renal transplants in the Middle East with special reference to histocompatibility matching, anti-rejection therapy with

ALG and prolonged preservation of imported cadaveric grafts. Annual Meetings of the Royal College of Physicians and Surgeons of Canada and the Canadian Transplantation Society, Calgary, Canada, September 1983.

4:41   Al Nakib W, **Abouna G M,** White A G, et al. Viral reactivation among renal transplant patients in Kuwait. The Third International Conference on the impact of viral diseases on the development of Middle East and African Countries, Kuwait, March 1983.

4:42   **Abouna G M,** White A G, Kumar M S A, Daddah S, Omar O F, Samhan M, John P & Kusma G. Experience with 100 consecutive living donor renal transplantations in Kuwait. Symposium on recent advances in Organ Transplantation, Ankara, Turkey, June 1983.

4:43   **Abouna G M,** White A G, Kumar M S A, Abbas A R & Soubky A S. Transplantation of imported kidneys from America and Europe with difficult problems and after prolonged preservation. Symposium on recent advances in Organ Transplantation, Ankara, Turkey, June 1983.

4:44   **Abouna G M.** Renal and pancreatic transplantation in diabetes. Diabetes Mellitus Update Symposium, Kuwait, February 1984.

4:45   **Abouna G M,** White A G, Kumar M S A, Daddah S K, John P, Omar O F & Silva O S G. Renal transplantation in Kuwait - Five years' experience. Second Kuwait International Medical Sciences Conference, Kuwait, March 1984.

4:46   Kumar M S A, White A G, **Abouna G M.** A trial of Cyclosporine - an immunosuppressive therapy in renal transplantation. Second Kuwait International Medical Sciences Conference, Kuwait, March 1984.

4:47   **Abouna G M,** Kumar M S A, Silva O S G, White A G, Daddah S & Samhan M. Successful transplantation longer than 50 hours by simple ice cooling. Second Kuwait International Medical Sciences Conference, Kuwait March 1984.

4:48   John P, Kumar M S A, White A G, Baissoni H, Silva O S G & **Abouna G M.** Living donors for kidney transplantation - a review of 130 consecutive donors. Second Kuwait International Medical Sciences Conference, Kuwait, March 1984.

4:49   Samhan M, Kumar M S A, White A G, Kusma G, Johnny K V & **Abouna G M.** Renal transplantation in paediatric recipients. Second Kuwait International Medical Sciences Conference, Kuwait, March 1984.

4:50   **Abouna G M,** Kumar M S A, White A G, Samhan M, Daddah S, John P, Silva S G & Soubky A S. Human cadaveric kidney preservation for periods greater than 50 hours: simple ice cooling versus hypotherm perfusion. The XIX Congress of the European Society for Surgical Research, Zurich, Switzerland, April 1984.

4:51 **Abouna G M,** Menkarious A, Baissoni H & Omar O F. Sugiura procedure versus portosystemic shunt operation for portal hypertension and bleeding varices. XIX Congress of European Society for Surgical Research, Zurich, Switzerland, April 1984.

4:52 Kumar M S A, White A G, Samhan M, Johny K V, Kusma G & **Abouna G M.** Donor specific transfusion (DST) in renal transplantation - is it worth it? Tenth Congress of the Transplantation Society, Minneapolis, MN, USA, August 1984.

4:53 **Abouna G M.** Living donor transplantation in the Middle East - experience with 145 recipients. Sixteenth International Course on Transplantation and Immunology, Lyon, France, May 1984.

4:54 **Abouna G M,** Menkarious A T, Baissoni H & Omar O F. Modified Sugiura procedure versus portosystemic shunt operations for portal hypertension and variceal bleedings. 45th Annual Meeting, British Society for Gastroenterology, Liverpool, UK, September 1984.

4:55 Kusma G, Kumar M S A, White A G, Samhan M, Johny K V & **Abouna G M.** Donor specific transfusion in renal transplantation. XXI Congress of the EDTA - European Renal Association, Florence, Italy, September 1984.

4:56 **Abouna G M.** Renal transplantation is best choice for treatment of renal failure. Update in Nephrology, Kuwait, January 1985.

4:57 **Abouna G M,** Kumar M S A, White A G, Samhan M & Daddah S A. Cyclosporine versus Azathioprine for immunosuppression in renal transplantation. Update in Nephrology, Kuwait, January 1985.

4:58 White A G, Kumar M S A & **Abouna G M.** Histocompatibility matching for renal transplantation in a single Centre. Update in Nephrology, Kuwait, January 1985.

4:59 Kumar M S A, White A G & **Abouna G M.** Prolonged preservation (30-76 hours) of imported human cadaveric kidneys. Update in Nephrology, Kuwait, January 1985.

4:60 **Abouna G M,** Menkarious A T, Baissoni H, Omar O F & Al Naqueeb B. Modified Sugiura procedure versus portosystemic shunt operations for portal hypertension and variceal bleeding - a prospective study. The Sixth Tripartite Meeting of the European Society for Surgical Research. The Society of University Surgeons (USA), and Surgical Research Society (UK), Boston, MA, USA, February 1985.

4:61 **Abouna G M.** Renal Transplantation - best alternative therapy for renal failure. Arab Health Conference, Dubai, UAE, February 1985.

4:62 **Abouna G M.** Coordination of kidney transplantation services within the Arab World. Arab Health Conference, Dubai, UAE, February 1985.

4:63 **Abouna G M,** Kumar M S A, White A G, Samhan M, Daddah S, John P & Silva O S G. Prolonged preservation of human cadaveric kidneys. What are the limiting factors? British Transplantation Society, Glasgow, UK, April 1985.

4:64 **Abouna G M.** Development of renal transplantation in Kuwait. International Conference on prospects of transplantation in Algeria, Algiers, Algeria, April 1985.

4:65 Kumar M S A, White A G, Silva S G & **Abouna G M.** Immunosuppression in preserved human cadaveric grafts - Azathioprine versus Cyclosporine A. International Conference on Prospects of Transplantation in Algeria, Algiers, Algeria, April 1985.

4:66 **Abouna G M.** Transplantation in Kuwait - Middle Eastern and North African perspective. Fist International Symposium on Renal Failure in Blacks, Washington, DC, USA, April 1985.

4:67 **Abouna G M.** The reversibility of diabetic nephropathy in man. The first International symposium on Renal Failure in Blacks, Washington, DC, USA, April 1985.

4:68 Kumar M S A, White A G, Silva S G & **Abouna G M.** Immunosuppression in pre-served human cadaveric grafts - Azathioprine versus Cyclosporine A. XXth congress of the European Society for Surgical Research, Rotterdam, Holland, May 1985.

4:69 **Abouna G M.** Kumar M S A, White A G, Samhan M, Daddah S, John P & Silva S G. Prolonged preservation in human cadaveric kidneys - what are the limits? XXth Congress of the European Society for Surgical Research, Rotterdam, Holland, May, 1985.

4:70 **Abouna G M,** Kumar M S A & White A G. Preservation of human cadaveric grafts for 30-76 hours. Annual Meeting of the Royal College of Physicians and Surgeons of Canada, Vancouver, Canada, September 1985.

4:71 **Abouna G M,** White A G, Kumar M S A & Silva S G. Cyclosporine versus Azathioprine in preserved human cadaveric grafts. Annual Meeting of the Royal College of Physicians and Surgeons of Canada, Vancouver, Canada, September 1985.

4:72 **Abouna G M.** Transplantation in the Middle East - problems and solutions. The First International Congress of the Middle East Dialysis and Organ Transplant Foundation, Istanbul, Turkey, November 1985.

4:73 Kumar M S A, White A G, Samhan M & **Abouna G M.** Experience with the transplantation of human cadaveric kidneys preserved for 30-76 hours. The First International Congress of the Middle East Dialysis and Organ Transplant foundation, Istanbul, Turkey, November 1985.

4:74 Kumar M S A, Samhan M, Daddah S, White A G & **Abouna G M.** Does the method of dialysis (hemo and peritoneal) affect the subsequent graft survival in renal transplant recipients? The First International Congress of the Middle East Dialysis and Organ Transplant foundation, Istanbul, Turkey, November 1985.

4:75 White A G, Kumar M S A, Strannegard O & **Abouna G M.** Renal transplantation in hepatitis 'B' surface antigen positive patients. The First International Congress of the Middle East Dialysis and Organ Transplant Foundation, Istanbul, Turkey, November 1985.

4:76 **Abouna G M,** White A G, Kumar M S A, Samhan M & Silva S G. Cyclosporine versus Azathioprine in preserved human cadaveric grafts. The First International Congress of the Middle East Dialysis and Organ Transplant Foundation, Istanbul, Turkey, November 1985.

4:77 **Abouna G M,** Kumar M S A & White A G. Optimum use of Cyclosporine in organ transplantation. Proceedings of the Symposium on the use of Cyclosporine in Clinical Transplantation, Cairo, Egypt, April 1986.

4:78 Kumar M S A, White A G, Samhan M S & **Abouna G M.** Cyclosporine in the treatment of acute renal allografts rejection. Proceedings of the International Symposium on Cyclosporine in Clinical Transplantation, Cairo, Egypt, April 1986.

4:79 Kumar, M S A, White A G, **Abouna G M,** & Samhan M. Non-related living donors for renal transplantation. XI International Congress of the Transplantation Society, Helsinki, Finland, August 1986.

4:80 White A G, Kumar M S A, Sanengard L R & **Abouna G M.** Renal Transplantation in hepatitis 'B' surface antigen positive patients. XI International Congress of the Transplantation Society, Helsinki, Finland, August 1986.

4:81 **Abouna G M,** Samhan M S, Kumar M S A, White A G & Silva S G. The limiting factors in prolonged preservation of human cadaveric grafts. XI International Congress of the Transplantation Society, Helsinki, Finland, August 1986.

4:82 **Abouna G M,** Sutherland D E R, Florack F, Heil J & Najarian J S. Preservation of human pancreatic allografts for 6-24 hours. XI International Congress of the Transplantation Society, Helsinki, Finland, August 1986.

4:83   Sutherland D E R, Goetz F, **Abouna G M**, & Najarian J S. Use of recipients' mesenteric (portal vessels) for revascularisation of human segmental pancreas grafts. XI International Congress of the Transplantation Society, Helsinki, Finland, August 1986.

4:84   Kalawi M, Kumar M S A, Panjwani D, Al Haf K, Shuwaikhi E & **Abouna G M.**   The epidemiology and prognosis of septicemia in renal transplant recipients. Third International Medical Science conference, Kuwait, March 1987.

4:85   Samhan M S. Kumar M S A & **Abouna G M.** Tuberculosis in renal transplantation. Third International Medical Science Conference, Kuwait March 1987.

4:86   Kumar M S A, Kalawi M, Araj G, Shakir R, Silva S G & **Abouna G M.** Listeria infection in renal transplant recipients. Third International Medical Science Conference, Kuwait March 1987.

4:87   **Abouna G M,** Heil J, Sutherland D E R & Najarian J. Factors necessary for successful 48 hour preservation of pancreas grafts. 13th Annual Meeting of the American Society of Transplant Surgeons, Chicago, USA, May 1987.

4:88   White A G, Kumar M S A, Silva S G, Al Shuwaikeh I & **Abouna G M.** Levels of ATP graft function in human cadaveric kidneys with prolonged cold ischemia. Fourth Annual Congress, European Society for Organ Transplantation, Gothenburg, Sweden, June 1987,

4:89   Panjwani D, Kumar M S A, Samhan M, White A G & **Abouna G M.** Graft loss due to chronic Cyclosporine toxicity in preserved cadaver grafts. Fourth Annual Congress, European Society for Organ Transplantation, Gothenburg, Sweden, June 1987.

4:90   Kumar M S A, White a G, Alex G, Antos M S, Philips E M & **Abouna G M.** Correlation of blood levels and tissue levels of Cyclosporine with the histologic features of Cyclosporine toxicity. Second International Congress of Cyclosporine, Washington, DC, USA, November 1987.

4:91   **Abouna G M,** Panjwani D, Kumar M S A, White A G, Al Abdullah I H, Silva O S G & Samhan M. The living unrelated donor - a viable alternative for renal transplantation. Third International Symposium on Organ Procurement, Barcelona, Spain, December 1987.

4:92   Samhan M, **Abouna G M,** Kumar M S A & Philips E M. Late function in 44 cadaver renal allografts preserved for 48-76 hours. Third International Symposium on Organ Procurement, Barcelona, Spain, December 1987.

4:93   **Abouna G M,** White A G, Al Abdullah I H, Kumar M S A, Panjwani D & Philips E M. The use of HLA mismatched living

140

related donors in renal transplantation is justified by the highly successful long-term results. Third International Symposium on Organ Procurement, Barcelona, Spain, December 1987.

4:94   **Abouna G M,** Samhan M & Kumar M S A. Unilateral native nephrectomy carried out through the same incision at time of renal transplantation is effective in the treatment of dialysis-resistant hypertension. Annual Meeting of the British Transplantation Society, Cardiff, UK, March 1988.

4:95   Kobryn A, Pasca A, White A G, Kumar M S A & **Abouna G M.** Are peripheral blood lymphocytes the source of elevated B-2 microglobulin in renal transplant recipients? 12th International Congress of the Transplantation Society, Sydney, Australia, August 1988.

4:96   Panjwani D D, Kalawi M, Kumar M S A, El Haj K, Araj G & **Abouna G M.** Septicaemia in renal transplant recipients: Epidemiology and prognosis. 12th International Congress of the Transplantation Society, Sydney, Australia, August 1988.

4:97   **Abouna G M,** Samhan M & Kumar M S A. Unilateral native nephrectomy at time of renal transplantation is effective in treatment of dialysis resistant hypertension. 12th International Congress of the Transplantation Society, Sydney, Australia, August 1988.

4:98   Kumar M S A, Samhan M, John P, Adnani M S & **Abouna G M.** Chronic Cyclosporine toxicity - is it the effect of preservation? 12th International Congress of the Transplantation Society, Sydney, Australia, August 1988.

4:99   Ruka M P, White A G, Kumar M S A, Al Abdullah I H & **Abouna G M.** Changes in the wet weight of pancreas during preservation in various solutions. 12th International Congress of the Transplantation Society, Sydney, Australia, August 1988.

4:100   Samhan M, Panjwani D, Al Dadah S, Kumar M S A, Araj G & **Abouna G M.** Tuberculosis: is it a contraindication to renal transplantation? 12th International Congress of the Transplantation Society, Sydney, Australia, August 1988.

4:101   Silva O S G, Shuwaikeh I, Shafei E, Hassan I M, Panjwani D, Kumar M S A & **Abouna G M.** Poor myocardial function in uremic patients improves significantly after renal transplantation. First International Congress of the Middle East Society for Organ Transplantation (MESOT), Ankara, Turkey, November 1988.

4:102   Samhan M, Kumar M S A, Silva O S G, Philips E M & **Abouna G M.** Renal transplantation in paediatric recipients. First International Congress of MESOT, Ankara, Turkey, November 1988.

4:103   **Abouna G M,** John P, Samhan M & Kumar M S A. Transplantation of single paediatric cadaveric kidneys into adult recipients. First International Congress of MESOT, Ankara, Turkey, November 1988.

4:104   Panjwani D, Sabawi N, White A G, Kumar M S A, Philips E M & **Abouna G M.** Existence of two distinct types of post renal transplant polycythemia - evidence from RBC mass studies. First International congress of MESOT, Ankara, Turkey, November 1988.

4:105   **Abouna G M.** Transplantation in the Middle East: problems and solutions. First International Congress of MESOT, Ankara, Turkey, November 1988.

4:106   Al Abdullah I H, Kumar M S A & **Abouna G M.** Prolongation of islets transplantation in outbred rats using Cyclosporine. First International Congress of MESOT, Ankara, Turkey, November 1988.

4:107   Al Abdullah I H, Kumar M S A & **Abouna G M.** Islets Transplantation in outbred rats using Cyclosporine. Second International Congress on Pancreatic and Islet Transplantation, Minneapolis, MN, USA, September 1989.

4:108   **Abouna G M,** Kumar M S A, Kalawi M, Samhan M, White A G, Al Abdullah I H, Kobryn A, Al Dadah S, Sabawi N, John P & Philips E M. Ten-year experience with 500 renal allografts in Kuwait. The Second International Congress of the Middle East Society for Organ Transplantation, Kuwait, March 1990.

4:109   Al Abdullah I H, Kumar M S A, Al Adnani M S & **Abouna G M.** Does pretreatment of islets of Langerhans with deoxyguanosine improve the islets survival without immunosuppression? The Second International Congress of the Middle East Society for Organ Transplantation, Kuwait March 1990.

4:110   White A G, Panjwani D, Angelo-Khattar M, Shihab Eldeen A, Kumar M S A, Philips E M & **Abouna G M.** Single Centre comparison of Cyclosporine assays and high pressure liquid chromatography. The Second International Congress of the Middle East Society for Organ Transplantation, Kuwait, March 1990.

4:111   Kalawi M, Al Sabawi N A, Samhan M, Panjwani D, Kumar M S A, Philips E M & **Abouna G M.** Cyclosporine withdrawal in renal transplant patients maintained on triple therapy. The Second International Congress of the Middle East Society for Organ Transplantation, Kuwait, March 1990.

4:112   White A G, Raju K T, Kumar M S A, Philips E M & **Abouna G M.** Rapid lymphocyte crossmatching for renal transplantation.

The Second International Congress of the Middle East Society for Organ Transplantation, Kuwait March 1990.

4:113   Al Dadah S, Kalawi M, John P, Abdul Karim H, Samhan M, Kumar M S A, Philips E M & **Abouna G M.** Review of 950 permanent vascular access procedures for hemodialysis. The Second International Congress of the Middle East Society for Organ Transplantation, Kuwait March 1990.

4:114   **Abouna G M.** John P, Kumar M S A, White A G, Silva O S G, Shuwaikhi E, Samhan M, Philips E M, Al Dadah S. Transplantation of small paediatric kidneys into adult recipients. The Second International Congress of the Middle East Society for Organ Transplantation, Kuwait March 1990.

4:115   Samhan M, Kumar M S A, Sabawi N, Silva O S G, Elzouki A Z, Al Dadah S, John P, White A G, Philips E M & **Abouna G M.** Renal transplantation in children. The Second International Congress of the Middle East Society for Organ Transplantation, Kuwait, March 1990.

4:116   **Abouna G M.** Values lost in commercialisation in organ transplantation - a Middle Eastern perspective. The Second International Congress of the Middle East Society for Organ Transplantation, Kuwait, March 1990.

4:117   **Abouna G M**, Kumar M S A, White A G, Samhan M, Kalawi M & al Sabawi N. Cyclosporine withdrawal in renal transplant recipients maintained on triple therapy. 13th International Congress of the Transplantation Society, San Francisco, USA, August 1990.

4:118   **Abouna G M.** The negative impact of paid organ donation. International Congress on Ethics, Justice and Commerce in Organ Transplantation, Munich, Germany, Dec 1990.

4:119   **Abouna G M,** Kumar M S A, Samhan M, et al. Transplantation of single paediatric kidneys into adult recipients. First International Congress of the Society for Organ Sharing, Rome, Italy, June 1991.

4:120   **Abouna G M,** Kumar M S A, Samhan M, et al. Preservation of kidneys longer than 48 hours. First International Congress of the Society for Organ Sharing, Rome, Italy, June 1991.

4:121   **Abouna G M.** Immunosuppression in renal transplantation. International Conference on Advances in Transplantation, Copenhagen, Denmark, March 1992.

4:122   **Abouna G M.** Shortage of donors for organ transplantation - possible solutions. Transplant Forum of the National Kidney foundation, Philadelphia, PA, March 1992.

4:123   **Abouna G M.** The successful utilization of kidneys with extended preservation and of paediatric kidneys for transplantation. TransLife Symposium on "The Marginal Donor", Orlando, FL, June 1992.

4:124   **Abouna G M.** Reversal of myocardial dysfunction in dialysis patients following successful renal transplantation. XIV International Congress of the Transplantation Society, Paris France, August 1992.

4:125   **Abouna G M.** The function of paediatric kidneys transplanted in adult recipients. The UNOS Region 2 Annual Meeting, Washington, DC, November 1992.

4:126   **Abouna G M.** Xenogeneic Baboon liver support as a bridge to liver transplantation in fulminant hepatic failure. The UNOS Region 2 Annual Meeting, Washington, DC, November 1992.

4:127   **Abouna G M.** Organ transplantation - future prospects. Presidential address given at the 3rd International Congress of the Middle East Society for Organ Transplantation, Tunis, Tunisia, December 1992.

4:128   **Abouna G M,** Kumar M S A, Miller J L, Rose L I, Brezin J, Chvala R, Lyons P, Katz S M & McSorley M. Combined kidney and pancreas transplantation from paediatric donors into adult recipients. Fourth International Congress on Pancreas and Islet Transplantation, Amsterdam, The Netherlands, June 1993.

4:129   Kumar M S A, Stephan R, Chui J, Chvala R P, Katz S M & **Abouna G M.** Donor age and graft outcome in cadaver renal transplantation. 2nd International Congress of the Society for Organ Sharing, Vancouver, British Columbia, July 1993.

4:130   **Abouna G M,** Kumar M S A, Chvala R P, Prior J E, Katz S M, Chui J & Samhan M. Experience in transplantation of paediatric kidneys into adult recipients. 2nd International Congress of the Society for Organ Sharing, Vancouver, British Columbia, July 1993.

4:131   **Abouna G M,** Kumar M S A, Chvala R, Brezin J, Lyons P & McSorley M. Transplantation of pediatric kidneys into adult recipients. XIIIth Annual Meeting of the North American Society for Dialysis and Transplantation, Maui, Hawaii, July to August 1994.

4:132   **Abouna G M.** Kidney transplantation from non-heart beating cadavers. TRENDS Cardiovascular and Trauma Conference, Philadelphia, PA, March 1994.

4:133   **Abouna G M,** Kumar M S A, Al Abdullah I H, Phillips K, Loose J & Sierka D. Induction immunosuppression with ATG in renal transplantation using variable dose according to the absolute CD3 T-Cell.

XIIIth Annual Meeting of the North American Society for Dialysis and Transplantation, Maui, Hawaii, July to August 1994.

4:134   **Abouna G M,** Kumar M S A, Chvala R & Curfman K. Kidney transplantation in patients older than 60 years of age - Is it worth it? Fourth International Congress of Middle East Society for Organ Transplantation (MESOT), Isfahan, Iran, October to November 1994.

4:135   Al Abdulla I H, Kumar M S A, Sullivan D K, Ilia H & **Abouna G M.** Auto transplantation of unpurified pancreatic islets of Langerhan into different sites in a canine model. Fourth International Congress of Middle East Society for Organ Transplantation (MESOT), Isfahan, Iran, October to November 1994.

4:136   **Abouna G M,** Kumar M S A, Chvala R, Brezin J & Samhan M. Transplantation of pediatric kidneys into adult recipients - A twelve-year experience. Fourth International Congress of Middle East Society for Organ Transplantation (MESOT), Isfahan, Iran, October to November 1994.

4:137   **Abouna G M,** Kumar M S A, Al Abdulla I H, Phillips K, Loose J & Sierka D. Induction immunosuppression with ATG in renal transplantation using a variable dose according to the CD3+ T Cells. Fourth International Congress of Middle East Society for Organ Transplantation (MESOT), Isfahan, Iran, October to November 1994.

4:138   Kumar M S A, Gridge P, Stephan R, Molavi A & **Abouna G M.** Infectious complications in the first 100 days after renal transplantation. Fourth International Congress of Middle East Society for Organ Transplantation (MESOT), Isfahan, Iran, October to November 1994.

4:139   **Abouna G M &** Al Abdulla I H. T-Cell and cytokine monitoring during ATG therapy in renal transplantation. First International Congress on Trace Elements, Tumour Markers and Cytokines, Kuwait University, Kuwait, March 1995.

4:140   **Abouna G M.** Current status of combined kidney and pancreas transplantation for diabetic neuropathy. IVth Congress of the Arab Society of Nephrology and Renal Transplantation, Tunis, Tunisia, April 1995.

4:141   **Abouna G M,** Al Abdulla I H & Ilia H. Plasmapheresis using human albumin or dectran 40 on the survival of pig to dog renal xenografts. Congress of the Society for Organ Sharing, Paris, France, July 1995.

4:142   **Abouna G M.** The negative impact of trading in human organs. IV World Congress of Surgery, Kiel Germany, September 1995.

4:143 **Abouna G M.** Current status of combined kidney and pancreas transplantation. Annual Congress of Lebanese Society of Nephrology and Transplantation, Beirut, Nov 1995.

4:144 **Abouna G M.** The Marginal Donors - Exploring the Outer Perimeters, 5th Congress of Middle East Society for Organ Transplantation, Cyprus, October 1996.

4:145 **Abouna G M.** Pancreas and Islet Cell Transplant for Treatment of Diabetes, 5th Annual Diabetic Conference of the Bahrain Diabetic Association Bahrain, December 1996.

4:146 **Abouna G M.** Ex-Vivo Xenogeneic Liver Support for Hepatic Failure - past, present and future. Medical Surgical Grand Rounds, University of Piza, Piza, Italy, January 1997.

4:147 **Abouna G M** & Hamdy H. Experience with new type of assessment for the MD examination - the Integrated Clinical Encounter Examination (ICEE). Association for Medical Education in Europe (AMEE), Conference on Teaching and Learning in Medicine, Vienna, Austria, September 1997.

4:148 **Abouna G M,** Hamdy H, El Shazali H, Tabbara K & Hassan K. Medical Education for the 21st Century: Experience at the Arabian Gulf University. 2nd Bahrain Arab American Conference & the 14th International Medical Conference of NAAMA. Manama, Bahrain, December 1997.

4:149 **Abouna G M,** Al Arrayed A S, Farid E, et al. Experience of Renal Transplantation in Bahrain. 2nd Bahrain Arab American Conference & the 14th International Medical Conference of NAAMA. Manama, Bahrain, December 1997.

4:150 **Abouna G M,** Al Arrayed A S, Farid E, et al. Mycophenolate Mofetil (MMF) Immunosuppression in high risk renal transplant recipients. 3rd International Conference on Immunosuppression. Geneva, Switzerland, February 1998.

4:151 **Abouna G M,** Ganguly P K, Hamdy H, et al. Ex-vivo liver perfusion system: An effective and successful method for hepatic support. Annual Congress of the British Transplant Society. Dublin, UK, April 1998.

4:152 **Abouna G M.** Artificial liver support for hepatic failure. Transplant Biology Research Centre & Massachusetts General Hospital, Harvard University, Boston, USA, May 1998.

4:153 **Abouna G M.** Changes in Medical Education at the Arabian Gulf University. Harvard Macy Institute Program for Leaders in Medical Student Education, Harvard Medical School, Boston, USA, May 1998.

4:154   **Abouna G M.** Hepatic support with ex-vivo liver perfusion. Beth Israel-Deaconess Medical Centre, Boston, USA, June 1998.

4:155   **Abouna G M.** Extracorporeal renal surgery and auto-transplantation of kidney, for reno vascular hypertension. Egyptian Association of Angiology & Vascular Surgery, 1st Arab World Meeting, Cairo, Egypt, June 1998.

4:156   **Abouna G M** & Hamdy H. The Integrated Direct Observation Clinical Encounter Examination (IDOCEE) - A reliable method of assessing student's clinical competence in problem based learning curriculum. 8th Ottawa International Conference, Philadelphia, USA, July 1998.

4:157   **Abouna G M.** Mycophenolate Mofetil Immunosuppression in high risk renal transplant recipients and Ex-vivo liver perfusion system: An effective and successful method for hepatic support. 27th World Congress of the Transplantation Society, Montreal, Canada, July 1998.

4:158   **Abouna G M** & Hamdy H. The Integrated Direct Observation Clinical Encounter Examination (IDOCEE) - A reliable method of assessing student's clinical competence in problem based learning curriculum. Association for Medical Education in Europe (AMEE) Annual Conference on Current issues in Medical Education, Prague, Czech Republic, Aug/Sept 1998.

4:159   **Abouna G M.** 'Extracorporeal xenogeneic liver perfusion system - A successful technique for hepatic failure as a bridge to liver regeneration or liver transplantation' and 'Comparison of plasmaphoresis using human albumin or Dextran-40 for removal of anti-gal xeno antibody in renal xeno transplantation'. 2nd International Exhibition and Conference of the INTERLAB98 - Laboratory Technology, Analysis, Diagnostics, Chemical Technology and Biotechnology, Cairo, Egypt, October 1998.

4:160   **Abouna G M.** Ex-vivo liver perfusion system for hepatic failure pending liver regeneation or liver transplantation. European Society of Artificial Organs, Bologna, Italy, November 1998.

4:161   **Abouna G M**, Al Arrayed A, Abdul A'al A, Tantawi M, Farid E. Experience of kidney transplantation in Bahrain: Medical, social and economic benefits. 1st GCC Medical Association Conference, Bahrain, November 1998.

4:162   **Abouna G M.** 'Medical Education for the 21st Century: Experience and Developments at the Arabian Gulf University' and 'Extracorporeal liver perfusion system for the treatment of patients with hepatic failure pending regeneration of their own liver or while awaiting liver transplantation'. 1st GCC Medical Association Conference, Bahrain, November 1998.

4:163   **Abouna G M.** 'Ex-vivo liver perfusion system for hepatic failure pending liver regeneration or liver transplantation'. American Hepato-Pancreato-Biliary Congress, Ft Lauderdale, Florida, USA, February 1999.

4:164   **Abouna G M.** Grand Round Presentations on 'Ex-vivo liver perfusion for hepatic failure: A controlled preclinical trial' at the University of Pennsylvania (Philadelphia), Rush Presbyterian St Lukes Medical Centre, North Western University (Chicago) and the University of Ottawa, February 1999

4:165   **Abouna G M.** 'Ex-vivo liver perfusion system for hepatic failure pending liver regeneration or liver transplantation' and Kidney transplantation from living donors - Medical and economic benefits and possible dilemmas'. Congress of Canadian Transplant Society, Alberta, USA, March 1999.

4:166   **Abouna G M, et al.** 'Ex-vivo liver perfusion - A successful method for support of patients in hepatic failure - Control Trial'. Annual Congress of the British Transplantation Society, Edinburgh, Scotland, March 1999.

4:167   **Abouna G M, et al.** 'Ex-vivo liver perfusion - A successful method for support of patients in hepatic failure - Control Trial'. Annual Congress of the American Society of Transplant Surgeons, Chicago, IL USA, May 1999.

4:168   **Abouna G M** "Medical Education for the Next Millennium" First Yemen-American Medical Conference, Sana, Yemen, October 26-30, 1999

4:169   **Abouna G M** "Current Status of Organ Transplantation", First Yemen-American Medical Conference, Sana, Yemen, October 26-30, 1999

4:170   **Abouna G M** "Marginal Donors – A Viable Solution for Organ Shortage", VII Congress of the Arab Society of Nephrology and Transplantation, Marrakech, Morocco, February 20-26, 2000

4:171   **Abouna G M** "The Humanitarian Aspects of Organ Transplantation", Invited Address at the Albert Schweitzer Gold Medal Award Ceremony, Warsaw, Poland, May 12, 2000

4:172   **Abouna G M et al.** "Ex-vivo Xenogenic Liver Perfusion System for Hepatic Failure Pending Liver Regeneration or Transplantation", VII Congress of the Middle East Society for Organ Transplantation, Beirut-Lebanon, June 7-11, 2000

4:173　**Abouna G M et al** "Ex-vivo Xenogenic Liver Perfusion System for Hepatic Failure Pending Liver Regeneration or Transplantation", XVIII International Transplantation Congress, Rome, Italy, Aug. 27-Sep 3, 2000

4:174　**Abouna G M et al** "Ex-vivo Xenogenic Whole Liver Perfusion System for Hepatic Failure Pending Liver Regeneration or Transplantation", XXII Surgical Congress, Athens, Greece, Nov 18-22, 2000

4:175　**Abouna G M et al** "Ex-vivo Liver Perfusion as a Bridge to Liver Regeneration or Transplantation", Canadian Society of Transplantation, Annual Congress, Lake Louise, Alberta Canada, March 17, 2001

4:176　**Abouna G M** "Sub-Optimal Donors as a Solution to Organ Shortage" and "Ex-Vivo Whole Liver Perfusion as a Bridge to Liver Transplantation or Liver Regeneration", 6th Congress of the International Society of Organ Sharing and Japanese Society of Organ Transplantation, Nagoya, Japan, July 22-27

4:177　**Abouna G M** "Sub-Optimal Donors as a Solution to Organ Shortage" and "Ex-Vivo Whole Liver Perfusion as a Bridge to Liver Transplantation or Liver Regeneration", 19th Annual Congress of South African Society of Organ Transplantation, Bloemfountein, S.A., September 16-20, 2001

4:178　**Abouna G M** "Sub-Optimal Donors as a Solution to Organ Shortage" and "Ex-Vivo Whole Liver Perfusion as a Bridge to Liver Transplantation or Liver Regeneration", 8th Congress Middle Eastern Society for Organ Transplantation, Muscat, Oman, October 21-24, 2002

4:179　**Abouna G M et al** "Ex-vivo Liver Perfusion as a Bridge to Liver Regeneration or Transplantation and Normothermic Preservation", 8th Congress Middle Eastern Society for Organ Transplantation, Muscat, Oman, October 21-24, 2002

National & International Scientific Meetings attended
Medical Centres visited & Postgraduate Courses taken
1968

- British Surgical Research Society Meeting, London, January 1968 (delivered a paper).
- British Surgical Research Society, Leeds, UK, July 1968 (delivered a paper).

- Annual Meeting of the Association of Surgeons of Great Britain. Royal College of Surgeons of England, April 1968 (delivered a paper for the Hoynihan Prize competition).
- Visited the Department of Surgery and the Transplantation Unit of the University of Cambridge, UK, February 1968 (Professor Roy Calne).

1969
- British Surgical Research Society Meeting, Oxford, UK, January 1969 (delivered 2 papers).
- Annual Meeting of the European Society of Clinical Investigation, Schevanegan, Holland, May 1969 (participated in a workshop on "Treatment of Hepatic Failure").
- Annual Meeting of the International College of Surgeons, Olympia, London, June 1969 (participant in Symposium on Liver Transplantation and Support Therapy).
- Annual Meeting of the European Dialysis and Transplant Association, Dublin, Ireland June 1969.
- International Symposium on Liver Support and Transplantation, Salzburg, Austria, April 1969 (participant).
- Annual Clinical Congress of the American College of Surgeons, San Francisco, October 1969.
- Visited the Department of Surgery and the Transplantation Service of the University of California, San Francisco, August 1969 (Professor Fred Belzer).

1970
- International Symposium on Organ Preservation, National Institute of Health, Bethesda, Maryland, Washington DC, April 1970.
- Visited the Transplantation Unit of the Medical College of Virginia, April 1970 (Professor David Hume).
- Annual Clinical Congress of the American College of Surgeons, Chicago, October 1970.

1971
- Annual Meeting of Society of University Surgeons, Hartford, Connecticut, February 1971.
- European Society for the Study of the Liver, Bern, Switzerland, August 1971.
- Third International Congress of the Transplantation Society, The Hague, September 1971 (delivered a paper).

1972
- International Symposium on Artificial Organ Support, New York, January 1972.Seventh Annual Congress of the European Society for Surgical Research, Amsterdam, April 1972 (delivered 2 papers).

- International Symposium on Organ Transplantation, Richmond, Virginia, May 1972.
- Fourth International Congress of the Transplantation Society, San Francisco, CA, September 1972 (participated in workshop on Hetero-transplantation).
- Visited the Department of Surgery, Stanford University Medical Centre, Stanford CA, September 1972 (Dr Robert Chase & Dr Norman Shumway).

1973
- Visited the Department of Surgery, Downstate Medical Centre, New York, January 1973 (Dr Sam Kuntz).
- Annual Meeting of Society of University Surgeons, New Orleans, Louisiana, February 1973.
- Eighth Congress of European Society for Surgical Research, Oslo, Norway, May 1973 (delivered 2 papers).
- Visited the Department of Surgery and Transplantation Service, University of Oslo, Norway, May 1973 (Professor Armesen & Dr Flatmark).
- Visited the Department of Surgery and Transplantation Surgery Unit, University of Edinburgh, Scotland, May 1973 (Sir Michael Woodruff).
- Annual Clinical Congress of the American College of Surgeons, Chicago, IL, October 1973 (delivered a paper).
- British Transplantation Society and the Society of Immunology, London, November 1973.

1974
- British Surgical Research Society, London, January 1974 (delivered a paper).
- British Transplantation Society and British Society of Immunology, London, April 1974.
- International Symposium on Hepatic Support, Kings College Hospital, London, September 1974 (invited participant).

1975
- Annual Meeting of the Royal College of Physicians and Surgeons of Canada, Winnipeg, Manitoba, January 1975 (delivered 2 papers).
- Tenth Annual Congress of the European Society for Surgical Research, Paris, April 1975 (delivered a paper).
- Visited the Department of Surgery, University of Lund, Lund, Sweden, April 1975 (Professor Stig Bengmark).

- Annual Meeting of the Canadian Medical Association, Calgary, Alberta, June 1975 (invited speaker).

1976
- Annual Meeting of the Royal College of Physicians and Surgeons of Canada, Quebec, January 1976.
- Workshop on Kidney Preservation, Cleveland Clinic, Cleveland, Ohio, May 1976 (invited participant).
- Sixth International Congress of the Transplantation Society, New York, August 1976 (delivered a paper).
- Postgraduate Course on "The Surgery of the Colon and Rectum", University of Minnesota, Minneapolis, November 1976.
- International Symposium on Artificial Organs, University of Strathclyde, Glasgow, Scotland, August 1976 (invited participant).
- Visited the Department of Surgery, University of Munich, Germany September 1976 (Professor Morer & Dr M Fischer).

1977
- International Conference on Fulminant Hepatic Failure. National Institute of Health, Bethesda, MD, March 1977 (invited participant).
- Twelfth Congress of the European Society for Surgical Research, Warsaw, Poland, April 1977 (Co-chairman for section on liver).
- Annual Meeting of the American Society of Transplant Surgeons, Chicago, May 1977.
- Postgraduate Course in Vascular Surgery, University of Minnesota, Minneapolis, June 1977.
- Postgraduate Course in "Controversial Areas in Surgery", Cleveland Clinic foundation, Cleveland, November 1977.

1978
- Postgraduate Course on GI Surgery, University of Minnesota, Minneapolis, June 1978.
- Visited the Department of Surgery, University of Minnesota, Minneapolis, June 1978 (Professors John Najarian, David Sutherland, Richard Buchwald).
- Annual Meeting of the European Society for the study of the Liver, Padova, Italy, August 1978.
- The International Congress of the Transplantation Society, Rome, Italy, September 1978 (delivered a paper).
- Annual Meeting of Society of Academic Surgery, Cleveland, Ohio, November 1978.

1979
- Annual Congress of European Society for Surgical Research, Barcelona, Spain, April 1979.

- European Dialysis and Transplant Association Annual Meeting Amsterdam, The Netherlands, June 1979.
- Symposium on Breast Cancer, University of Nottingham, England, July 1979.
- Annual Meeting of the British Society of Oncology, Nottingham, July 1979.
- Tripartite Meeting of British SRS, the European SSR and the Society of University Surgeons, Oxford, July 1979.6.   Postgraduate Course in Surgery, Massachusetts General Hospital, Boston, October/ November 1979.

1980
- Attended International Congress of the Transplantation Society, Boston, June/July 1980 (participated in the symposium on anti-lymphocyte globulin in treatment of allografts rejection).
- Attended British Surgical Research Society Meeting, Nottingham, July 1980. Attended Annual Clinical Congress of the American College of Surgeons, Atlanta, Georgia, October 1980.

1981
- Attended International Medical Exhibition, Dubai, February 1981.
- 9th Annual Symposium on Vascular Surgery of Society of Clinical Vascular Surgeons, Palm Springs, April 1981.
- 18th Annual UCLA Seminar on Controversial areas in Surgery, Palm Springs, April 1981.
- Annual Meeting of American Society of Transplant Surgeons, Chicago, June 1981.
- Visited the Department of Surgery, Northwestern University, Chicago, June 1981 (section of vascular surgery, Dr John Bergan).
- Visited the Department of Surgery, Section of Transplantation, University of Minnesota, July 1981 (Drs Najarian, Sutherland & R Simmons).
- 18th Congress of European Dialysis and Transplant Association, Paris, July 1981.
- Visited the University of Claud-Bernard, Lyon, France, Section of Transplantation and Nephrology, July 1981 (Professors Traeger & Dubernard).
- International Congress on Chemotherapy, Florence, Italy, July 1981.
- International Vascular Symposium, Royal Festival Hall, London, September 1981.

- Euro-transplant Annual Meeting, Leiden, Holland, September 1981.
- Annual Clinical Congress of American College of Surgeons, San Francisco, CA, October 1981.

1982

- International Symposium on Vericeal Bleeding, Royal Society, London, January 1982.
- Symposium on Cancer Education, Kuwait, January 1982 (Session Chairman & participant).
- First International symposium on the Surgery of the Alimentary System, Kuwait, February 1982 (Chairman of Organising Committee, Session Chairman & Speaker).
- Third Meeting of Arab Board for Surgical Specialties, Doha, Qatar, March 1982.
- International Urology Symposium, Dubai, UAE, March 1982 (invited speaker).
- International Symposium on Plasmapheresis, Cleveland Clinic, Cleveland, OH, April 1982.
- Visited the Departments of Clinical Surgery and Surgical Research of University of Munich for one week to discuss the new technique of extra-corporeal destruction of renal stones by shock waves and problems relating to renal and pancreatic transplantation, April 1982.
- Seventh Saudi Medical Congress, Dammam, Saudi Arabia, May 1982 (by invitation).
- Eighth Annual Meeting of the American Society of Transplant Surgeons, Chicago, IL, June 1982.
- External Examiner, King Saudi University, Riyadh, Saudi Arabia, June 1982.
- Study leave for two months (July to September 1982) working on Bone Marrow Transplantation at the Fred Hutchinson Cancer Research Center in Seattle, WA (Dr E Thomas) and the John Hopkins Bone Marrow Transplant Programme, Baltimore, MD (Dr George Santos); and also Pancreas Transplantation at the University of Minnesota, Minneapolis, (Drs John Najarian & David Sutherland).
- Attended the 9th International Congress of the Transplantation Society, Brighton, UK, August 1982. Attended the 7th congress of the International Microsurgical Society, Lyon, France, September 1982.
- Attended the 68th Annual Congress of the American College of Surgeons, Chicago, IL.
- External Examiner for FRCS, Royal College of Surgeons of Ireland, Dublin, Ireland, November 1982.

1983

- Mediterranean Netilmicin Symposium, Nice, France, February 1983 (Chairman of Session & Speaker).
- Visiting Professor, University of Baghdad, Iraq, February 1983.
- International Congress on Organ Procurement, Maastricht, The Netherlands, April 1983 (Chairman of Session & Speaker).
- First International Congress on Cyclosporine, Houston, TX, May 1983.
- Participated in the First International Congress on Transplantation in Diabetics, The Hague, The Netherlands, September 1983.
- Visiting Surgeon - Liver Transplantation Service, University of Pittsburgh, Pittsburgh, PA, September 1983 (Dr Thomas E Starzl). Assisted at seven liver transplant operations as well as donor hepatectomy, and participated in the follow-up of some 25 patients recently transplanted.
- Participated in the Annual Meeting of the Royal College of Physicians and Surgeons of Canada, Calgary, Alberta, September 1983 (presented a paper).
- Attended the 69th Annual Clinical Congress of the American College of Surgeons, Atlanta, GA, October 1983.

1984

- Postgraduate Symposium in GI Surgery, Kuwait, January 1984 (speaker).
- International Symposium on Diabetes Mellitus Update, Kuwait, February 1984 (speaker).
- XIX Congress of the European Society for Surgical Research, Zurich, Switzerland, April 1984 (speaker).
- 16th International Course on Transplantation and Immunology, Lyon, France, May 1984 (speaker).
- 10th Annual Meeting of the American Society of Transplant Surgeons, Chicago, IL, June 1984.
- 10th Annual Meeting of the Transplantation Society, Minneapolis, MN, August 1984.
- Clinical Congress of the American College of Surgeons, San Francisco, CA, October 1984.

1985

- Arab Health Conference, Dubai, UAE, February 1985.
- Conference Sur La Transplantation Renale, Algiers, Algeria, April 1985.
- First International Congress on Renal Failure in Blacks, Washington, DC, April 1985.

- Annual Meeting of the Arab Board of Surgery, Damascus, Syria, April 1985.
- Annual Congress of the European Society for Surgical Research, Rotterdam, Holland, May 1985.
- Annual Meeting of the American Society of Transplant Surgeons, Chicago, IL, May 1985.Visited the Department of Surgery, University of Wisconsin Medical Centre to observe and discuss their program of hepatic and pancreatic transplantation and their experimental work in organ preservation, August 1985 (Drs F O Belzer, Hans Sollinger & Munci Kalayogly).
- Visited the Mayo Clinic, Rochester MN, to observe and discuss their hepatic transplantation programme, August & September 1985 (Drs Kreom & Weizner).
- Visited the Fred Hutchinson Cancer Centre, Seattle, WA to observe and discuss developments in bone marrow transplantation, September 1985 (Drs Donald Thomas, Rainer Storb & Keith Sullivan).
- Annual Meeting of the Royal College of Physicians and Surgeons of Canada, Vancouver, September 1985.
- The Second International Symposium on Organ Procurement and Preservation, Detroit, MI, October 1985.
- First International Congress of the Middle East Dialysis and Transplant Foundation, Istanbul, Turkey, November 1985.

1986
- Visited the Department of Surgery, Rush-Presbyterian/St Luke's Medical Centre, Chicago, IL to observe and discuss their experimental and clinical liver transplant programme, January 1986 (Dr James Williams).
- Visited the Department of Surgery, University of Nebraska Medical Centre, to observe and discuss their hepatic transplantation programme, February 1986 (Dr Byers Shaw & Rikkers).
- Postgraduate Symposium on Liver Diseases, Kuwait University, February 1986. (Participant & Main Speaker).
- Annual Meeting of the American Society of transplant Surgeons, Chicago, IL, May 1986.
- The XI International Congress of the Transplantation Society, Helsinki, Finland, August 1986.
- The 72nd Clinical Congress of the American College of Surgeons, New Orleans, LA, October 1986.
- The International Mediterranean Congress of Chemotherapy, Cairo, Egypt, October 1986.

1987
- Attended the Round Table Conference on the Clinical use of OKT-3 for the Treatment of Allograft Rejection, Paris, France, February 1987.
- Annual Meeting of the American Society of Transplant Surgeons, Chicago IL, May 1987.
- Annual Clinical Congress of the American College of Surgeons, New Orleans, La, October 1987.

1988
- First International Congress on Pancreatic and Islet Transplantation, Stockholm, Sweden, March 1988.
- XII International Congress of the Transplantation Society, Australia, August 1988 (Chairman of Session).
- Annual Meeting of the American Society of Transplant Surgeons, Chicago, IL, June 1988.
- First International Congress of the Middle East Society for Organ Transplantation, Ankara, Turkey, November 1988.
- Annual Congress of the American College of Surgeons, Chicago, IL, October 1988.

1989
- 15th Annual Scientific Meeting, American Society of Transplant Surgeons, Chicago, IL, May 1989.
- Ethics, Justice and Commerce in Transplantation: A global view, Ottawa, Canada, August 1989 (Chairman of session).
- Visiting Surgeon, Liver Transplant Service, University of Chicago (Dr C Broelsch) and the University of Nebraska, Omaha (Dr B Shaw) July-August 1989.
- 4th International Congress on organ procurement and preservation and the Second International Congress on Pancreas Transplantation, Minneapolis, MN, September 1989 (Chairman of Session).
- Clinical Congress of the American College of Surgeons, Atlanta, GA, October 1989.
- Middle East Medicare Conference and Exhibition, Bahrain, October 1989 (Chairman of Session).
- 4th Congress of the European Society of Organ Transplantation, Barcelona, Spain, October 1989.

1990
- Second International Congress of the Middle East Society for Organ Transplantation, Kuwait City, March 1990 (Chairman of Congress).
- Annual Meeting of the American Society of Transplant Surgeons and the American Society of Transplant Physicians, May-June 1990.

- Visited the Section of Liver Transplantation of the University of Chicago to participate in the new procedure of surgical liver transplantation from related donors, Chicago, IL, July 1990 (Dr C Broelsch).
- The 13th International Congress of the Transplantation Society, San Francisco, CA, August 1990 (Co-chairman of Session).
- Second International Congress on Peri-operative Liver Transplant Care, Pittsburgh, PA, September 1990.
- International Congress on Ethics, Justice and Commerce in Organ Replacement Therapy, Munich, Germany, December 1990 (invited speaker).

1991

- United Network for Organ Sharing (UNOS), Atlanta, GA, February 1991.
- Conference on Organ Transplants in Children - A Perspective for the 90's, St Christopher's Hospital for Children, Philadelphia, Pa, April 1991.
- American Society for Artificial Internal Organs, Chicago, IL, April 1991.
- Annual Meeting of the American Society of Transplant Surgeons and the American Society of Transplant Physicians, Chicago, IL, May-June 1991.
- Society for Organ Sharing, Rome, Italy, June 1991.
- Visiting Surgeon at the Clinical Pancreas Transplant Programme, University of Minnesota, Minneapolis, MN, July 1991 (Dr David E R Sutherland).
- First International Congress on FK506, Pittsburgh, PA, August 1991.
- First International Congress on Xenotransplantation, Minneapolis, MN, August 1991.
- Bowel Transplant Meeting, London, Ontario, October 1991.
- European Society for Organ Transplantation, Maastricht, The Netherlands, October 1991 (Chairman of Scientific Session).
- Annual Meeting of the American College of Surgeons, Chicago, IL, October 1991.

1992

- Annual Meeting of the United Network for Organ Sharing (UNOS), Washington, DC, February 1992.
- International Conference on Advances in Transplantation, Copenhagen, Denmark, February 1992 (invited speaker).
- Transplant Forum of the National Kidney Foundation, Philadelphia, PA, March 1992.

158

- Second International Symposium on Liver Transplantation, Minneapolis, MN, April-May 1992.
- University of Wisconsin, Madison, WI, May 1992 (Visiting Professor).
- Meeting of the American Society for Artificial Internal Organs, Nashville, TN, May 1992.
- Annual Meeting of the American Society of Transplant Surgeons, Chicago, IL, May 1992.
- First International Congress of the Cell Transplant Society, Pittsburgh, PA, May 1992.
- National Symposium on the Marginal Donor, Orlando, FL, June-July 1992 (invited speaker).
- XIV International Congress of the Transplantation Society, Paris, France, August 1992.
- Annual Meeting of the Canadian Royal College of Surgeons, Ottawa, Ontario, September 1992.
- Annual Meeting of the American College of Surgeons, New Orleans, LA, October 1992.
- UNOS Region 2 Annual Meeting, Washington, DC, November 1992 (speaker).
- Third International Congress of the Middle East Society for Organ Transplantation, Tunis, Tunisia, December 1992 (President of the Society and invited speaker).

1993
- Transplantation conference of the US Department of Health and Human Services, Public Health Service, Arlington, VA, February 1993.
- Foreign Relations Committee of UNOS, Chicago, IL, March 1993 (acting Chairman).
- Annual Meeting of the American Society of Transplant Surgeons, Houston, TX, May 1993.
- IVth International Congress on Pancreas and Islet Transplantation, Amsterdam, the Netherlands, June 1993 (presented a paper).
- Visiting Professor, Kuwait University, June 1993
- Second International Congress of the Society for Organ Sharing, Vancouver, British Columbia, July 1993 (Chairman of Scientific Session).
- Second International Congress on Xenotransplantation, Cambridge, UK, September 1993.
- Annual Meeting of the International Liver Transplantation Society, Toronto, Ontario, October 1993.

- American College of Surgeons 79th Annual Clinical Congress, San Francisco, CA, October 1993.
- Laparoscopic Cholecystectomy Course, Ethicon. The Endo-Surgery Institute, Cincinnati, OH, November 1993.

1994

- International Congress on New Trends in Immunosuppression, Geneva, Switzerland, February 1994.
- Symposium on Reno-Vascular Hypertension - Current Diagnosis and Treatment, Pennsylvania Hospital, Philadelphia, PA, March 1994.
- Second International Congress of the Cell Transplant Society, Minneapolis, May 1994 (presented a paper).
- American Society of Transplant Surgeons, Annual Congress, Chicago, May 1994.
- Annual Meeting of North American Society for Dialysis and Transplantation, Maui, Hawaii, July 1994 (presented papers).
- Workshop on "Problem Based Learning" McMaster University, Faculty of Health Sciences, Hamilton, Ontario, Canada, October 1994.
- Workshop on "The McMaster System of Undergraduate Medical Education" and visits with Dean, Associate Deans of Education and other Faculty, McMaster University, Faculty of Health Sciences, Hamilton, Ontario, Canada, November 1994.

1995

- International Congress on Trace Elements, Tumour Markers and Cytokines, Kuwait University, March 1995 (invited speaker).
- IVth Congress of Pan African and Pan Arab Societies of Nephrology and Transplantation Tunis, Tunisia, April 1995 (invited speaker).
- External Examiner in Surgery, Kuwait University, June 1995.
- Congress of the International Society for Organ Sharing, Paris, France, July 1995.
- IVth World Congress of Surgery, Kiel, Germany, September 1995 (invited speaker).
- Lebanese Society for Dialysis and Transplantation, Beirut, Lebanon, October 1995 (invited speaker).
- Meeting of the Deans of Medical Schools in the GCC Countries, "The Medical Curriculum at AGU", Muscat, Oman, October 1995.

- Autumn Meeting of the British Transplantation Society, London, England, November 1995.

1996

• Invited by a number of Universities in Northern Italy, Modena, Ferrara, Trieste, Milan and Torino as Visiting Professor in order to help them in their program of establishing an artificial liver support device as a bridge to liver transplantation, January 1996 (Dr G Costa).

• Italian Artificial Liver Support Consortium of the Universities of Milan, Pisa, Modena and Trieste, February 1996.

• 3rd Arab League Conference on Arabisation of Medical Education, Kuwait City, Kuwait, April 1996.

• 6th Congress of the International Association of Middle East Studies, Amman, Jordan, April 1996.

• 42nd Annual Conference of the American Society for Artificial Internal Organs (ASAIO), Washington, May 1996.

• International College of Surgeons, Convocation Ceremony at the 58th Annual Meeting of the US Section, Washington DC, May 1966.

• Current Controversies in Vascular Surgery Workshop, Harvard Medical School, Boston, May 1996.

• External Examiner, Kuwait University, June 1996.
• 7th International Ottawa Conference on Medical Education and Assessment, Maastricht, Holland, June 1996.

• Invited as Visiting Professor to assess progress on Liver Support Apparatus, Universities of Modena and Milano, Italy July 1996.

• Invited Guest, University of Pittsburgh's, Starzl Transplant Institute, USA August 1996.

• 16th International Congress of the Transplantation Society, Barcelona, Spain, August 1996.

• Invited as Visiting Professor and Advisor for Liver Transplantation Programme, Universities of Milano, Modena and Pisa, Italy October 1996.

- 82nd Annual Clinical Congress of the American College of Surgeons (ACS), San Francisco, USA, October 1996.

- 5th Congress of the Middle East Society of Organ Transplantation (MESOT), Limassol, Cyprus, October 1996.

- Invited to review the Liver Support Machine, Universities of Milano, Modena and Piza, Italy December 1996.

1997

- Invited as Visiting Professor to supervise the multicentre trial of the Liver Support Apparatus, Universities of Pisa, Italy, January 1997.

- Invited to participate in the International Business Communications Conference, Tolerance & Immunotherapy in Allotransplantation Conference, San Diego, USA, February 1997.

- 4th GCC Medical Deans Meeting, Kuwait University, April 1997.

- 23rd Annual Scientific Meeting of the American Society for Transplant Surgeons (ASTS), Chicago, USA, May 1997.

- External Examiner, Department of Surgery, Kuwait University, June 1997.

- 4th International Congress of the Society of Organ Sharing, Washington, USA, July 1997.

- The Association for Medical Education in Europe (AMEE), Teaching and Learning in Medicine, Vienna, Austria, September 1997. (Speaker & Chairman of session)

- 8th Congress of the European Society for Organ Transplantation (ESOT), Budapest, Hungary,
  - September 1997. (Invited)

- 4th International Congress of Xenotransplantation, Nantes, France, September 1997.

- 83rd Clinical Congress of the American College of Surgeons, Chicago, USA, October 1997.

- 6th International Congress of the Arab Association of Pediatric Surgeons, Manama, Bahrain, October 1997. (Keynote Speaker)

- 5th GCC Medical Deans Meeting, Riyadh, Saudi Arabia, October 1997.

- Arab Nephrology and Renal Transplant Society, Beirut, Lebanon, November 1997. (Keynote Speaker)

- 2nd Bahrain Arab American Conference & 14th International Medical Conference NAAMA (National Arab American Medical Association), Manama, Bahrain, December 1997. (Speaker & Chairman of Session)

1998

- Meeting of the Multi Centre Trial on the Abouna/Costa Liver Support Machine, Mirandola, Italy, February 1998 (Invited to participate and Chair the meeting).

- 3rd International Conference on New Trends in Clinical and Experimental Immunosuppression, Geneva, Switzerland, February 1998. (Invited)

- New Dimensions in Transplantation Conference, Florence, Italy, February 1998. (Invited)

- Annual Congress of the British Transplant Society, Dublin, UK, April 1998. (presented a paper)

- 6th GCC Medical Deans Council Meeting, Al Ain, United Arab Emirates, May 1998. (Chairman)

- Transplant Biology Research Centre and Massachusetts General Hospital Harvard University, Boston, USA, May 1998 (Invited Speaker).

- Harvard Macy Institute program for "Leaders in Medical Student Education", Harvard Medical School, Boston, USA, June 1998 (Invited Participant).

- Beth Israel-Deaconess Medical Centre, Division of Transplantation, Boston, USA, June 1998 (Invited Speaker).

- University of Kuwait Medical College, Kuwait, June 1998 (External Examiner in Surgery).

- Egyptian Association of Angiology & Vascular Surgery, 1st Arab World Meeting, Cairo, Egypt, June 1998 (Invited Guest Speaker).

- 8th Ottawa International Conference, Philadelphia, USA, July 1998 (Presenter).

- 27th World Congress of the Transplantation Society, Montreal, Canada, July 1998.

- Association for Medical Education in Europe (AMEE) Annual Conference on Current issues in Medical Education, Prague, Czech Republic, Aug/Sept 1998 (Presenter).

- INTERLAB'98 2nd International Conference on Biotechnology, Cairo Egypt, October 1998 (Invited Guest Speaker)

- Annual Congress of the American College of Surgeons, Orlando, Florida, USA, October 1998.

- European Society of Artificial Organs, Bologna, Italy. November 1998 (Presenter).

- University of Kuwait Medical College, Kuwait, December 1998 (External Examiner in Surgery).

1999

- American Hepato-Pancreato-Biliary Congress, Ft Lauderdale, Florida, USA, February 1999.

- Congress of Canadian Transplant Society, Alberta, USA, February 1999.

- Grand Round Presentations at the University of Pennsylvania (Philadelphia), Rush Presbyterian St. Lukes Medical Centre, North Western University (Chicago) and the University of Ottawa, February & March 1999.

- 20th Anniversary Celebration of Starting Transplantation in Kuwait, Invited speaker and honored by Kuwait Ministry of Health (March 1999)

- British Transplantation Society, Edinburgh, Scotland, March 1999. (Presenter)

- American Society of Transplant Surgeons May 1999 (Presenter)

- Invited speaker at the 1st Yemen American Medical Conference Sani, Yemen Oct. 1999

- University of Kuwait College of Medicine Nov. 8, Dec 9, 1999 (Visiting Professor)

2000

- Visiting Professor and invited speaker, New York Medical College, NY (Jan 2000)

- Invited Speaker at the 6th Congress of Arab Society of Nephrology and Renal Transplantation, Marrakech, Morocco (Feb 2000)

- Invited Speaker at the University of Calgary Medical Center, Foothills Teaching Hospital, Calgary, Alberta Canada (Apr 2000)

- The Annual Congress for the American Society of Transplantation 2000, Chicago, IL, USA May 13-18, 2000

- Invited Speaker at and recipient for the presentation of the Albert Schweitzer Gold Medal for Medicine for the year 2000, Polish Academy of Medicine, Warsaw, Poland, May 12, 2000

- Middle East Society for Organ Transplantation, VII Congress, Beirut-Lebanon, June 7-11, 2000 (Invited Speaker)

- XVIII International Transplantation Society Congress, Italy, Rome, Aug 27-Sep 3, Invited Presenter

- The Annual Congress of the American College of Surgeons, October 23-27, 2000, Chicago, IL, USA

- XXII Panhellenic Surgical Congress, November 18-22, 2000, Athens, Greece, (Invited Speaker)

2001

- Canadian Society of Transplantation, March 15-18, 2001, Annual Congress, Lake Louise,
    Alberta, Canada

- American Society of Transplantation, May 11-16, 2001, Annual Congress, Chicago, IL, USA

- 6th Congress of the International Xeno Transplantation Association, September 29-Oct 3, 2001 Chicago, IL, USA

- Conference on Transplant Immunosuppression, Minneapolis, MN, USA October 24-27, 2001

- 5th Congress of the Turkish Society of Transplantation, November 6-9, 2001 Ankara, Turkey

2002

- American Society of Transplant Surgeons (ASTS), Winter Symposium, January 25-28, 2002, Miami, FL

- American Society of Transplant Surgeons (ASTS), April 26 – May 1, 2002, Washington, DC

- 8th Congress of the International Liver Transplant Society, June 12-15, 2002, Chicago, IL

- 8th Congress of the Middle East Society for Organ Transplantation (MESOT), October 21-26, 2002, Muscat, Oman

2003

- American Society of Transplant Surgeons (ASTS), Winter Symposium, January 24-26, 2003, Miami, FL

- American Hepato-Pancreato Biliary Assoc Congress, February 27-March 2, 2003, Miami, FL
- Canadian Society of Transplantation Congress, March 20-23, 2003, Lake Louise, Alberta Canada

- British Transplant Society Annual Congress, April 8-10, 2003, London UK

- American Society of Transplantation Congress, May 30-June 4, 2003, Washington, D.C

- Turkisk Transplantation Society and Euro Transplantation Joint Congress, Ankara, Turkey, June 24-24, 2003
- 7th Congress of International Society for Organ Donation and Procurement, November 27 – December 1, 2003, Warsaw, Poland

2004

- American Society of Transplantation Congress, Winter Symposium, January 22-25, 2004, Scottsdale, Arizona, USA
- 7th Annual Congress of British Transplantation Society, April 28-30, 2004, Birmingham, UK

About the Author

Dr. Johna is an Assyrian physician born and raised in the suburbs of Baghdad, Iraq. He graduated form the University Of Baghdad College Of Medicine in 1983. After six years of active duty in the Iraqi military during the first and the second Gulf Wars, he migrated to the United States of America where he finished a residency in general Surgery. He joined the faculty at Loma Linda University School of Medicine where he is currently serving as an Associate Clinical Professor of Surgery. In addition to his interest in clinical research and surgical education, he is interested in the history and culture of his battered nation. In addition to this book, he published The memoirs of Allen Oldfather Whipple: The Man Behind the Whipple Operation. tfm publishing, London, 2003, and Twenty-Five Years in Persia: The Memoirs of Mary Allen Whipple. 1stBooks Library, Indiana, 2003.

Printed in the United States
24196LVS00004B/244-261

9 781418 480608